FIT FOOD FOR FELLAS

Virginia Hill

Lothian
BOOKS

Acknowledgements

Recipe development by Jodie Hollands
and Bianca Stafrace

Thomas C. Lothian Pty Ltd
11 Munro Street, Port Melbourne, Victoria 3207

First published 1997
Reprinted 1998

National Library of Australia
Cataloguing-in-Publication data:

Hill, Virginia– .
Fit Food for Fellas

Includes index.
ISBN 0 85091 858 8.

1. Cookery (Natural foods). 2. Quick and easy cookery.
I. Title.

641.563

Cover and text design by Jo Waite
Illustrations by Denica Wapshott
Cover photographs by Lynette Zeeng
Typesetting by Figment
Kitchen tools courtesy of Minimax Pty Ltd;
tool belt attachments courtesy of D. & J. Evans
Printed by Australian Print Group

CONTENTS

INTRODUCTION

'Kissing don't last: cookery do!'

— George Meredith (1859).

An evening spent with the young players of the Collingwood Footy Club, teaching some cooking basics for their survival skills off the field, left me wondering why, after twenty-five years of women's liberation, mothers had failed to teach their sons how to be involved with food in any way, except to eat it!

This lack of first-hand learning has led to two generations of Australians who cannot cook, simply because they do not know simple cooking techniques and rarely buy raw ingredients, despite the diversity of produce in supermarkets nationally. Paradoxically, men have always dominated cooking in the public arena, but, beyond the barbecue, blokes today do not know how cooking works and are often intimidated by recipe writers who assume readers know what the cooking process is all about!

As one of my older male colleagues remarked, 'I've gone from Hell's kitchen to a dream kitchen, and I still can't cook anything because recipes are so rigid and do not use words like toss, shake and stir. Let's face it, what does "Cook until done" mean?' With this in mind, I have developed recipes using up to six easy and accessible ingredients, with generally only two or three simple cooking steps to explain what to do, so you too can give cooking a go.

Use the recipes as a starting point; they are not prescriptions. Check out what food you have on hand, what you can make from it, and the seasonality of fresh food so it is available and cheap. Taste the food while you are cooking, and then adjust it to your taste — a liberating experience that should encourage you to move on to the 'short-order ideas' in different sections of the book.

Dining in is to be respected in an era when more than a quarter of the household's weekly food budget is spent on eating outside the home (emulating Americans' fast-food choices), and we have now become the second-most-obese race after the United States of America! As a result, we are not a pretty sight, or the healthy nation we should be.

Follow the fit tips to ensure you eat well, live longer, and enjoy an active sex life. Whether through necessity or desire you need to cook, view it as an opportunity to be fearless, flamboyant and messy if you like (it's your kitchen, and you have to clean it) while destressing from the daily disciplined grind.

Eating together informally or formally is important for social wellbeing, enjoyment, conversation and socialising with your family, friends or business associates.

Don't hesitate to mix and match the recipes in the book to suit yourself and the ingredients you already have. Vegies, meat and herbs are versatile.

Before you cook any of the recipes, check that you have all the ingredients (See the sample shopping list on page 13), then assemble all the ingredients and utensils ready to go.

So here's to comfort, confidence and cheer in your kitchen.

P.S. A serious message for any 'significant female other' in the household:

'Some of us have become the men we wanted to marry' — Gloria Steinem.

Keep out of the kitchen while the fellas are cooking. Everyone cooks differently, and while their procedures may not be 'right' according to your way of doing things, enjoy the nurturing aspect of eating food someone else has prepared.

Fitness File

Here are some suggestions for you to help cut back on the fat in your diet and keep your weight in check without having to stick to an unworkable health regime.

- Use non-stick cookware. There are some excellent quality frypans and saucepans available in supermarkets. They hold the heat well, and clean easily, and they require little or no fat for cooking.
- Read food labels carefully — 'light' may not mean low-fat. All Australian food lists the ingredients, with the most prominent ingredient first, followed by the next major ingredient, and so on. Limit any commercially prepared food where fat is included as one of the first three ingredients in the list.
- Heat a small amount of oil in the pan before you add the other ingredients, as hot oil is thinner and will go further.
- Use an oil spray for your frypan or wok. Minimise the amount of fat by spraying lightly.
- Marinades do not have to contain oil, and will increase the flavours of skinless chicken, fish and meat (page 92).
- Keep your knives sharp, making it quicker and easier to trim fat from meat and poultry (page 8).
- Use small amounts of packet stocks instead of fat to cook onions and garlic.
- Make oil-free dressing by combining vinegar and your favourite mustard.
- Turn yoghurt into a light mayonnaise by adding some mayonnaise and a pinch of curry.
- Try some of the low-fat dairy products for a healthier choice. They are rich in protein and calcium.
- Rev up a smoothie with low-fat milk and frozen fruit (page 181).
- Snack on popcorn, it is nearly fat-free (page 131).

Essential Kitchen Gizmos

Knives, stainless steel: 1 small
Knives, stainless steel: 1 large
Chopping boards (wooden)
Cup measure
Measuring spoons
Scales
Potato peeler
Grater
Tongs (for the oven or BBQ)
Oven gloves or pot holders
Whisk (or fork)
Egg lifter
Soup ladle
Carving fork and knife
Colander (for pasta or vegetables)
Mesh strainer (for draining liquid or fat)
Blender (for blending drinks and dips)
Can opener
Lemon juicer
Mixing bowls

Optional extras

Wooden spoon
Slotted spoon
Knife sharpener
Mallet (for pounding meat)
Icecream scoop (or spoon)

Cookware for Fitness

Non-stick frypan
Wok
Non-stick small and large saucepans, and lids
Metal baking tray (preferably non-stick) or a foil baking tray as a substitute
Cake pan

Microwave Modcons

Microwave-safe containers, with a lid

Small (0.7–1 litre), for vegetables, sauces, scrambled eggs
Medium (1.5 litres), for soups, reheating rice or pasta, casseroles
Large (2.25 litre), for soups, one-pot dishes, cakes
4 cup (1 litre) ovenable glass jug, for custards, soups and rice

Always select the right-sized container for the amount of food being cooked to allow room for the food to sit comfortably or expand (especially when making cakes).

If you do not have a turntable in your microwave oven, rotate the food one-third of a turn three times during the cooking time.

Ovenproof glass cookware is suitable for use in both microwave and conventional ovens, and can go from oven to table.

Microwave accessories

- Plastic wrap may be used in place of a lid on a variety of containers. Check that it is marked 'microwave safe' so that it will withstand the high temperature of steam.

  Venting: leave a space at the edge of the container or jug to allow steam to escape from under the plastic wrap, and to prevent food from boiling over during cooking.
- Non-recycled plain white paper towel is recommended (but not recycled paper towel, which may contain metal fragments that can ignite or cause arcing in the oven). Use this towel over foods (such as roast beef) to absorb excess moisture and to prevent spattering in the oven.

- Baking paper serves as a non-absorbent lining for containers, or as a parcel for meals cooked in the microwave (or conventional oven) to retain moisture.
- Aluminium foil can be used for shielding meat or fish to prevent overcooking. The rule of thumb is a ratio of 70 per cent food to 30 per cent foil. Ensure that no foil touches the oven walls, as this will cause sparking, a reaction known as arcing, which can damage the oven walls because of the intense heat produced.

Disposables

Baking paper (to cover the oven tray and to save washing up)
Cling wrap (to cover the microwave dishes)
Foil (to keep food warm)
Paper towel, non-recycled (for draining fat from foods or to use in the kitchen in place of a teatowel; to cook on in the microwave oven, or to cover microwave dishes)

Stocking Up

Kitchen cupboard

A well-stocked kitchen cupboard is the key to quickly bringing together a good meal or snack, so make sure you have the right basic ingredients on hand to make a quick and delicious meal with the minimum effort.

Check the following list, and stock up with items you are likely to use regularly.

- Rolled oats, natural muesli, rice bran, All-bran
- Multigrain bread, brown bread with added grains, pocket pita bread, mountain bread
- Muffins, crumpets, Ry Vita, Weet-Bix
- Popcorn
- Water biscuits
- Pasta: spaghetti, spaghettini, fettucine, penne, shells, vegeroni, wholemeal pasta, couscous, Asian noodles
- Rice: white and Quick Brown Rice
- Pulses: lentils, split peas, kidney beans
- Dried herbs (see page 14) and spices

Cans

- Baked beans, chick peas, butter beans, bean mixes, kidney beans
- Tomatoes, sweetcorn kernels, asparagus (low-salt varieties)
- Evaporated low-fat milk, skim-milk powder
- Apricots, mangoes, passionfruit, peaches, pears, pineapple, in natural fruit juice

Dried fruit

- Sultanas, raisins, currants, dates, fruit medley, fruit salad

Oils

- Olive oil, olive or canola oil cooking spray

Dressing

- Vinegar, balsamic vinegar

Miscellaneous

- Nuts: unsalted peanuts, pecans, walnuts and pine nuts
- Seeds: pumpkin (pepitas) and sesame seeds
- Bottled sundried tomatoes and peppers, Thai curry paste, pesto (keep refrigerated when opened)

Fridge and freezer

- Fish
- Eggs
- Lean beef, pork, lamb, skinless poultry
- Fresh herbs: parsley, basil or coriander (they will keep for a week in a jar of water covered with a plastic bag)
- Canola margarine
- Low-fat milk
- Natural low-fat yoghurt, low-fat flavoured fruit yoghurt
- Cheeses: smooth ricotta, Parmesan, mozzarella, low-fat cheddar, cottage cheese, cheese slices
- Fresh fruit and vegetables
- Frozen vegetables and berries
- Low-fat icecream

Front Foot in the Kitchen

- Keep your hands clean with soap and water. Always wash your hands before handling any food.
- Use paper towel to clean up splashes on the floor (not the sponges or dishcloths).
- Paper towels are for hands, and are disposable; teatowels are for drying dishes, and need washing regularly.
- Keep work surfaces clean, and wipe them down with a cleaner after use.
- Keep chopping boards scrupulously clean; wash immediately after use. Scrub the boards well, as strong flavours like onion, garlic and chilli transfer.
- Wash dishes and pan immediately after use. If you are fortunate enough to have a dishwasher, rinse plates, etc., if you are not putting it on immediately.
- Keep perishable foods cold until required.
- Cover foods to be refrigerated.
- Do not reheat foods more than once.
- Take care if others are using the kitchen at the same time (especially children), when using sharp implements, or when transferring hot foods or boiling liquids.
- Keep some first aid handy.
- Do not leave hot fat or oil unattended.
- Keep a fire mat or extinguisher in the kitchen, and install a smoke alarm.

Know Your Knives

Cook's knife: an all-purpose knife, with a broad blade; it is curved from blade to tip.

Utility knife or kitchen knife: a smaller version of the cook's knife.

Serrated knife or slicing knife: this knife has a rigid blade with scalloped edges and a blunt tip, and is used for slicing bread and tomatoes.

Cleaver: it has a rectangular blade favoured by Asian chefs because it is versatile, good for smashing garlic, and for chopping through meat and bones.

Carving knife: this knife has a long, thin, flexible blade, which easily slices through meat or poultry.

Knife knacks

- A sharpening steel is a must for keeping your knives sharp.
- Hang your knives on a magnet bar or in a knife block to protect the blades. Keep all knives out of the reach of small children.
- It is best to cut on a thick wooden chopping board, as cutting on marble or its equivalent will blunt your knives.
- Wash and dry your knives immediately after use.

Cooking Guidelines

All the recipes in this book give the combined preparation and cooking times for both conventional and microwave methods, so whichever one you choose you will know how long you will need to spend in the kitchen. Select the menu for your meal according to a comfortable time allowance. Remember, you can mix and match recipes to make the meal of your choice (or according to the ingredients you have available).

Microwave cooking

Microwave ovens cook by power and not heat, which makes them clean, convenient and easy to use for many of the recipes in this book.

To ensure that you have success with your recipes, here are some guidelines to familiarise you with the principles of microwave cooking.

Timing

The weight of the food determines the length of cooking time in the microwave oven. The more food you cook at one time, the longer it takes (the amount of microwave energy that can be absorbed is reduced when the total quantity of food is increased).

The rule of thumb is to multiply the original cooking time by the increased amount of food, then subtract slightly to prevent overcooking, for example,

Chicken fillets	*Minutes*
1	3
2	6 – 1 = 5
3	9 – 2 = 7

Size

Small pieces of food cook faster than large ones. To cook food evenly, cut all the pieces to the same size.

Shape

Evenly shaped pieces of food cook best. Irregularly shaped foods (like pears or lamb racks) take longer to cook in the thicker parts. To cook them evenly, place the thickest portion at the outer edge of the container to receive the maximum amount of energy (microwaves work in straight lines from the outside of the food to the inside).

Starting temperature

Food to be cooked in the microwave should be at room temperature: the colder the food at the start of cooking, the longer it takes to heat. Cooking times for this book are calculated at room temperature.

Fat and bone content

Microwaves are attracted to fat, and fat cooks more quickly than meat — thin layers of fat on a rack of lamb will speed cooking. Lean meat is recommended in the recipes, so remove all visible fat.

Bone is an excellent conductor of heat, and can cause the surrounding meat to overcook. Boneless cuts of meat cook more evenly.

Density

Different densities of food affect the ease of microwave penetration. Porous foods like tomatoes will cook faster than potatoes, which are dense, although the foods may be the same size.

Standing time

Some cooking will continue within microwaved food after the energy source is turned off, or after the food is removed from the oven, because of the heat stored inside the food itself.

Rest the food after cooking time to allow for this extra cooking. This standing time will vary, but can be estimated as approximately a quarter of the total cooking time.

Microwave power settings

Power level settings control the percentage of microwave energy able to enter the oven.

Power level (%)	*Microwave heat*	*Conventional heat*
10–20	WARM	Cool
30–35	DEFROST	Slow
30–40	LOW	Moderately slow
50–60	MEDIUM	Moderate
70–80	MEDIUM–HIGH	Moderately hot
90–100	HIGH	Hot

Conventional cooking: oven temperatures

Celsius (°C)	*Fahrenheit (°F)*	*Description*
110	225	Very cool
120	250	
140	275	Cool
150	300	
160	325	Moderate
180	350	
190	375	Moderately hot
200	400	
220	425	Hot
230	450	
250	475	Very hot

Standard metric measurements

1 cup	250 ml
1 tablespoon* (tbsp)	20 ml
1 teaspoon* (tsp)	5 ml

** All spoon measurements are level.*

Food measurements

	Weight (g), 1 metric cup
Bread and cereals	
breadcrumbs:	
soft	60
dry	125
flour:	
cornflour	130
white, plain or self-raising	125
wholemeal, plain or self-raising	135

	Weight (g), 1 metric cup
pasta (e.g. penne)	150
rolled oats, uncooked	90
rice:	
brown or white, uncooked, short grain	210
brown or white, uncooked, long grain	200
Dried fruit	160
Meat alternatives	
dried beans	200
dried peas	185
dried split peas or lentils	200
nuts, chopped	125
Dairy products	
cheese, grated	125
yoghurt (1 carton)	200
Miscellaneous	
sugar:	
brown, firmly packed	170
white, castor	225

	Weight (g), 1 level tbsp
butter or margarine	20
cornflour	10
custard powder	10
honey	30
nuts, chopped	10
sugar	15

Quick Reference to Cooking Terms

The cutting edge

Chop	Cut into cubes or slices of no particular size, but keep even in size.
Chop finely	Cut into tiny pieces.
Cube	Cut food into cubes about 2 cm across, larger than dice.
Dice	Squares of food, smaller than a cube.
Grate	Rub food (e.g. cheese) over a flat or convex grater to give coarse or fine threads.
Shred	Cut food into narrow strips.
Slice	Cut thin broad pieces of food 2–3 mm thick.

Cooking commands

Blend Mix foods together to achieve a smooth consistency. A technique used in the preparation of sauces, soups and casseroles.

Cover Use of a lid, foil or plastic wrap to keep food moist and to prevent it from boiling down during cooking.

Done To tell when foods such as cakes and desserts (e.g. cheesecake) are cooked, insert a skewer into the centre to see if it is soft or set. The skewer should be clean when removed.

Pound Beat food such as meat and poultry with a mallet to achieve an even thickness and to prevent toughening during cooking.

Simmer Cook food in liquid just below the boiling point.

Stir Agitate ingredients gently with a spoon during cooking to ensure the heat is distributed equally, so the mixture is smooth. This action also helps to prevent sticking and burning.

Toss Turn over the leaves of salad to make sure they are evenly coated with dressing, preferably just before serving.

Whisk Use a kitchen utensil (made of stainless steel wire bent into loops, with a handle) or a fork to beat and emulsify mixtures so that they will not be lumpy.

When Disaster Strikes

1 Review the problem.
2 Resurrect the good portion.
3 Place in a clean utensil.
4 Decide if the food can be revived and extended by adding more of a basic ingredient. For example:
   - boilovers, such as custard — try adding milk, and beating vigorously.
   - burning — if possible, trim and discard the outside burnt edges, slice the food, and reheat in a sauce over gentle heat or in a microwave oven on MEDIUM (50%) for 2–5 minutes.
   - sticking to the base of containers — remove the usable food, and check to see if it will blend with cooked rice or pasta, or canned beans. Stir it through, and call it a casserole.

Fast-track Shopping Tips

- Most people don't like shopping, so the quickest and most efficient place to go is a good local supermarket. It pays to shop at the end of the day when you can buy reduced-price goods from the fresh-food counters. Be sure to use these items quickly.

- If you have time and are looking for really fresh food at competitive prices, head for your local market, especially just before closing time when prices are at rock bottom (check the *Yellow Pages* for outlets). Buy seasonally — that is, when certain fruits and vegies are available from local producers.
- Try teaming up with friends to shop at bulk stores for pantry ingredients.
- Make a shopping list — and stick to it. Shop once a week if possible, at the least crowded time, to save time and money.
- Avoid shopping when you're hungry so you will not be tempted to buy ready-made, high-fat, fast-fix foods.
- Try to shop without the anklebiters, and you won't be tempted to fill the trolley with their (your) favourite food.
- Become an accomplished cook — that way you won't be tempted to buy ready-to-go, high-fat dish meals as you'll know how to cook your own favourites.

Eating well is easier than you think!

Sample Menu and Shopping List

Chicken Balls over Gnocchi and Tomato

200 g lean chicken mince
2 tbsp breadcrumbs
1 tbsp plum sauce
1 tsp dried basil (or 1 tbsp fresh basil, chopped)
1 (55 g) egg
½ cup flour
1 (370 g) jar Italian Tomato Pasta Sauce
1 (625g) pkt gnocchi (cooked)

Fresh Berries with Vitari Ice

Shopping List

Grocery

Breadcrumbs, 250 g pkt
Plum sauce, 250 ml bottle
Dried basil, small pkt (or fresh, see Fruit and vegetables, below)
Flour, plain, 1 kg pkt
Italian Tomato Pasta Sauce, 370 g jar

Meat and poultry

Chicken mince, 200 g pkt

Deli and dairy

Eggs, 6 (55 g)
Gnocchi, 625 g pkt
Vitari Ice Confection, 250 g carton

Fruit and vegetables

Basil, fresh 1 bunch (or dried, see Grocery, above)
Strawberries, blueberries or raspberries, 250 g

Form Guide for Herbs

Try some aromatherapy in your food.

Basil: best with Italian dishes, tomato and pasta dishes.

Chives: a relative of the onion, and a tasty addition to omelettes, potato and green salads.

Coriander or Chinese parsley: gives a spicy flavour to Asian food, especially Thai dishes.

Parsley: a good all-rounder; it blends well with other herbs and seasonings, and is great on pasta or rice dishes, or mixed in with minced meat.

Mint: traditionally served with lamb, but good with other savoury salads, e.g. cucumber and yoghurt (page 78).

Rosemary: an aromatic herb for lamb, chicken or fish; especially good when barbecuing or roasting these meats.

All these herbs can be purchased in a 'freshly bottled' form in the supermarket, and keep well for months in the fridge.

Note: 1 tbsp fresh herbs = ½ tsp dried herbs

Pesto

Pesto is a robust and addictive herb sauce for pasta or minestrone. It is easily made in a blender (see page 152).

Breakfast for Champions

'I grew up eating Vita Brits and it was a real challenge for me to build up to 14, to give me more energy'

— Trevor Hendy, Ironman.

Breakfast is always a challenge, given the time of day and the amount of time left to eat it, which is often dependent on the previous evening's entertainments!

Fit Tips

- Any champion knows that you cannot win the race if you miss the start! Eating a healthy breakfast is the only way to start the day properly Not only will it boost your blood-sugar levels, and maximise your energy levels and concentration over the day, but breakfast helps to boost your metabolism, which is great for keeping body-fat levels under control.
- Research has shown a much lower incidence of industrial accidents for people who eat breakfast.

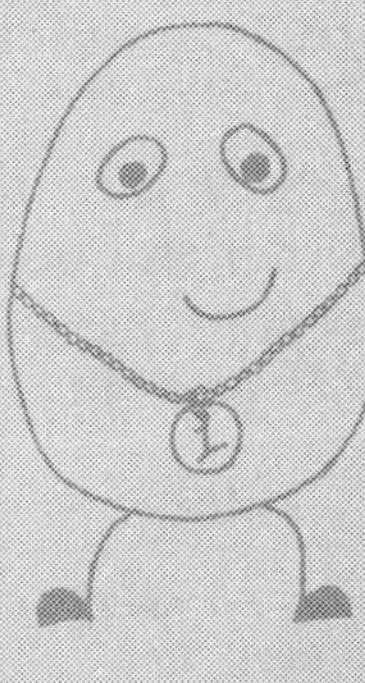

Daily Double

Ironman Bricks (page 22)
Mango and Passionfruit Booster (page 22)

This winning combination of cereal and lean meat with a drink packed with Vitamin C provides over 90% of your daily iron needs, and a massive 45% of your daily Vitamin C requirements!

Power Breakfast

Dried-fruit Fix (page 23)
Muesli Yoghurt Deuce (page 24)
Egg and Bacon Towers (page 25)

A high-carbo breakfast with a hefty punch of protein. Great for blokes who are bulking up or who have jobs with high-energy needs.

Gut Cruncher

Crunchy Grapefruit (page 26)
Meaty Mushroom Omelette (page 27)

Your abdominal region will benefit more from what goes into your mouth than how many sit-ups or crunches you do at the gym. A high fibre intake helps keep food moving efficiently through your gut, so reducing the risk of bowel disorders such as cancer, constipation, diverticulitis and irritable bowel syndrome.

Slam-dunk Breakfast

Manpower Milkshake (page 28)
Big-flavour Bubble 'n' Squeak (page 65)

Drinks are a great way to have a quick breakfast, particularly if you make them the night before, then slam them down as you leave for work or school. You can blend almost any fruit into a milkshake for a high-carbohydrate, high-calcium, low-fat breakfast. You would struggle to find a healthier option than vegetables on toast to finish!

Breakfast Trifecta

V8 Heart Starter (page 28)
Mustard Scrambled Eggs in One (page 29)
Toast Toppers (page 30)

The first 'leg' of this breakfast will wake you up, the second will provide protein for power, and the third 'leg' will give you enough energy for much more than a day at the races!

How to Cook Eggs

Eggs are quick and easy to prepare, and lend themselves to preparation by both conventional and microwave cooking.

As eggs cook very quickly, take care not to overcook them. Most dishes should be removed from the heat just before completion of cooking, as the heat within the dish will continue the cooking process.

Boiled Egg

Most people do not know how to boil an egg properly. This method ensures the yolk is in the centre, and that the eggshell does not crack.

Serves 1

1 (55 g) egg
water
pinch of salt
1 slice of wholegrain toast

CONVENTIONAL (5–8 MINUTES)

pin
small saucepan
slotted spoon

1 PIERCE the round end of the eggshell with a pin to allow the air to escape.
2 BRING a small saucepan of water to the boil, and add a pinch of salt.
3 LOWER the egg gently into the water, and boil for 3–5 minutes.

Remove egg with a slotted spoon, and serve with toast.

For a hard-boiled egg, cook for a further 8 minutes, then plunge it into cold water to prevent a dark ring forming around the yolk.

MICROWAVE (1 MINUTE)

small cup
fork
plastic wrap

1 PLACE 1 tbsp water in a small cup.
2 BREAK the egg carefully into the cup, and prick the yolk with a fork to prevent the egg from exploding.
3 COVER with plastic wrap, and cook on HIGH (100%) for 30–40 seconds until white is just set.

Serve the egg with toast.

Poached Egg

SERVES 1

1 (55 g) egg
water
slice of wholegrain toast

frypan
cup
slotted spoon

CONVENTIONAL (4–5 MINUTES)

1 PUT 2 cm cold water in the frypan, and bring to a simmer over medium heat.
2 BREAK the egg into a cup or saucer, and carefully pour into the water.
3 COOK the egg for 3–4 minutes until the white is set. Remove with the slotted spoon, and drain well.

Serve on toast.

HANDY MAN HINTS

- *Another way to make toast if you do not have a toaster: place the bread slices underneath a hot griller until the bread turns brown; then cook the other side.*
- *To test the freshness of an egg, hold it up to the light — a very small air chamber indicates a fresh egg.*

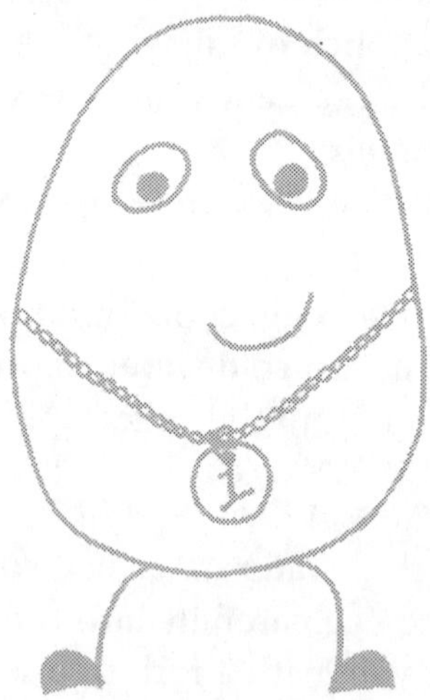

Scrambled Eggs

Gentle heat and gentle mixing are what make really creamy scrambled eggs.

SERVES 1

2 (55 g) eggs (allow 2 eggs per person)
2 tbsp low-fat milk
salt and pepper, or a pinch of dried mixed herbs
1 tsp butter or margarine

CONVENTIONAL (5 MINUTES)

fork
small bowl or jug
heavy-based saucepan
wooden spoon

1 BEAT the eggs and milk together with a fork in a small bowl or jug, adding a little seasoning.
2 MELT the butter or margarine in a heavy-based saucepan over low heat, and pour in the eggs (too much heat will make the eggs leathery).
3 STIR slowly and continuously with the wooden spoon until the egg mixture is thick and creamy. Remove the pan from the heat just before the eggs are thoroughly cooked.

Serve immediately on toast.

MICROWAVE (2 MINUTES)

fork
small bowl or jug
plastic wrap
spoon

1 BEAT the eggs, milk and seasonings together with the fork in the small bowl or jug.
2 COVER with plastic wrap, and cook on HIGH (100%) for 1 minute. Stir.
3 COVER, and cook on HIGH (100%) for a further 30 seconds.

Stir, and serve immediately on toast.

Omelette

SERVES 1

2 (55 g) eggs
2 tbsp water (for microwave method use milk)
1 tsp butter or margarine
filling of your choice (see hint below)

CONVENTIONAL (5 MINUTES)

small bowl or jug
fork
non-stick frypan
tablespoon
teaspoon
egg lifter

1 LIGHTLY beat the eggs and water together with a fork in a small bowl or jug.
2 PREHEAT the frypan until it is very hot. Place the nob of butter or margarine in the pan. Allow to melt, then pour in the egg mixture.
3 DRAW the cooked egg mixture from the edges towards the centre of the pan with a spatula, tilting the pan to allow uncooked mixture to flow underneath the edges. Continue until the mixture no longer flows.

Fill one side of the omelette, and fold before serving.

MICROWAVE (3–4 MINUTES)

teaspoon
plain dinner plate
small bowl or jug
fork
tablespoon
egg lifter

1 PLACE the knob of butter or margarine on a dinner plate, and cook on HIGH (100%) for 30 seconds.
2 BEAT the eggs and milk together with the fork in the small bowl or jug, and pour onto the plate. Cover with unvented plastic wrap, and cook on MEDIUM–HIGH (70%) for 1 minute.
3 LIFT the cooked egg, allowing any uncooked egg mixture to flow underneath the edges. Cover, and cook on MEDIUM–HIGH (70%) for 1–1¼ minutes. Allow to stand for ½ minute.

Fill one side of the omelette, and fold before serving.

HANDY MAN HINT

Fillings for the omelette are limited only by your imagination: you could use shredded lean chicken or ham or low-fat cheese; sliced tomatoes and chopped spring onions. The filling should be at room temperature (the heat of the omelette is sufficient to warm the filling) and if necessary precooked (e.g. bacon).

Fried Egg

Serves 1

1 (55 g) egg
½ tsp oil
1 slice wholegrain toast

teaspoon
non-stick frypan
spatula

CONVENTIONAL (4 MINUTES)

1 HEAT the frypan over low heat, and cover the base of the pan with the oil.
2 BREAK the egg carefully into the pan. Cook gently for about 3 minutes, basting continuously, turning the egg over halfway through the cooking time.

Serve immediately on toast.

MICROWAVE (1 MINUTE)

custard cup or
small soufflé dish
or small plate
skewer or toothpick
plastic wrap

1 PLACE the oil in the custard cup or dish. Cook, uncovered, on HIGH (100%) for 30 seconds.
2 BREAK the egg into the cup or dish, and prick the egg yolk and white. Cover, and cook on HIGH (100%) for 30 seconds.

Serve immediately on toast.

Cooking times for microwave dishes are approximate, because the time will vary according to egg size, temperature of the egg, and the oven wattage.

HANDY MAN HINT

For a fast fried egg, cook until the white has set but do not turn the egg over.

Ironman Bricks

Serves 1

6 Weet-Bix
80 g light cream cheese
1 medium-sized tomato, sliced
100 g lean ham, sliced

CONVENTIONAL (5 MINUTES)

1 SPREAD cheese over three Weet-Bix, and cover this with the tomato and ham.
2 TOP with the remaining Weet-Bix.

Serve with a sprig of fresh basil.

chopping board
serrated knife
2 plates
table knife

HANDY MAN HINT *Light cream cheese spreads easily. These snacks are good for morning tea or after work.*

Mango and Passionfruit Booster

Serves 1

1 cup orange juice
1 (170 g) can passionfruit pulp
1 (450 g) can mango slices
ice (optional)

CONVENTIONAL (2 MINUTES)

1 PLACE all the ingredients, except the ice, in a blender. Blend for 30 seconds.
2 POUR over the ice in the glass.

Serve immediately.

cup measure
can opener
spoon
blender or fork
long glass

HANDY MAN HINT *If you do not have a blender, mash the mango slices with a fork. Combine all the ingredients in a screwtop jar, and shake vigorously.*

FIT TIP *Use fresh juice.*

VARIATION *Turn this into a mint julep by placing crushed ice and mint leaves in a tall glass, and pour the mango–passionfruit blend over the ice. Decorate with a few fresh mint leaves.*

Dried-fruit Fix

SERVES 2

300 g mixed dried fruit of your choice (apricots, apples, sultanas, mixed fruit, raisins, peaches, etc.)
1 cup apple juice
2 tbsp sugar
½ cup water
1 tsp vanilla

CONVENTIONAL (14–18 MINUTES)

1 COMBINE all the ingredients in the saucepan. Stir over medium heat for 6–8 minutes until the sugar is dissolved.
2 COVER, and simmer over medium heat for a further 8–10 minutes, stirring once.

Serve warm or cold, with low-fat yoghurt or icecream.

scales
wide-based saucepan, and lid
wooden spoon
cup measure
tablespoon
teaspoon
serving bowl

MICROWAVE (8 MINUTES)

1 COMBINE all the ingredients in the microwave-safe container. Cover, and cook on HIGH (100%) for 4 minutes.
2 STIR. Cover, and cook for a further 4 minutes.

Serve warm or cold, with low-fat yoghurt or icecream.

scales
medium-sized microwave container, and lid
wooden spoon
cup measure
tablespoon
teaspoon
serving bowl

HANDY MAN HINT

Keep the fruit salad in the fridge, and use over cereal or yoghurt for a great power breakfast.

Muesli Yoghurt Deuce

SERVES 2

2 cups natural muesli
2 cups low-fat milk
2 (200 g) tubs low-fat fruit yoghurt
2 bananas, sliced

CONVENTIONAL (5 MINUTES)

2 bowls
spoon
cup measure
chopping board
small knife

1 PLACE 1 cup muesli and 1 cup milk in a bowl, and top with half of the yoghurt.
2 REPEAT with the remaining ingredients.

Serve, topped with banana slices.

HANDY MAN HINT

A medium-sized banana contains as much fibre as 1½ slices of wholemeal bread, and is totally fat free. Use a sliced banana as a toast topper.

FIT TIP

Reduced-fat milk and yoghurt have more protein and calcium than full-cream varieties.

Egg and Bacon Towers

Serves 2

2 (55 g) eggs
4 rashers lean rindless bacon (150 g)
1 (130 g) can baked beans (salt reduced)
4 slices wholemeal bread, toasted
35 g low-fat cheddar cheese, sliced

CONVENTIONAL (10 MINUTES)

can opener
spoon
non-stick frypan
egg lifter or fork
chopping board
knife
paper towel
plate

1 HEAT the frypan over medium heat, crack the eggs into the pan and cook over medium heat for 1 minute until they are firm and set. Turn the eggs, and cook for a further minute. Remove the eggs from the pan onto a warmed plate.
2 COOK the bacon over high heat for 4–5 minutes (turning occasionally) or until the rashers are browned and crisp. Remove from the pan and drain on paper towel; place on the warm plate beside the eggs. Drain and wipe the pan. Add the baked beans, and heat for 2 minutes.
3 PLACE one slice of toast on a plate, cover with one cooked egg, half the bacon and cheese, and half the baked beans. Top with another slice of toast.

Repeat for the second serve.

HANDY MAN HINTS

- *Warm plates by placing a little water on each plate and microwave on HIGH (100%) for 30 seconds for each plate. Alternative method: place plates in the sink and cover with the hot water; leave for several minutes, then drain.*
- *Keep sliced bread in a plastic bag in the freezer, and use as required.*

FIT TIP

Fat does not make you full. Recent research at the University of Sydney found that people who ate a high-fat breakfast were hungrier and ate more for lunch than those who ate the same amount of kilojoules in carbohydrates. If you are starving by lunchtime, try eating more carbohydrates for breakfast (e.g. cereal, bread, fruit).

Crunchy Grapefruit

Serves 2

2 grapefruit, halved (4 halves)
4 tbsp honey
½ cup natural muesli
4 strawberries

2 bowls
serrated knife
1 tablespoon
cup measure

CONVENTIONAL (5 MINUTES)

1 PLACE the grapefruit halves in the bowls. Run a knife inside the edge of each grapefruit between the skin and the flesh, and between each segment to loosen them.
2 DRIZZLE the honey over the grapefruit halves, and sprinkle with muesli.

Serve with each half topped with a strawberry.

HANDY MAN HINT

Heat honey in its jar: remove the metal lid, and heat the jar in the microwave oven on HIGH (100%) for one minute to make the honey run easily.

Meaty Mushroom Omelette

Serves 2

1 tbsp olive oil
2 spring onions, chopped
5 mushrooms, sliced (150 g)
40 g sundried tomatoes, chopped
4 (55 g) eggs, lightly beaten
1 tbsp fresh parsley, chopped, or ½ tsp dried parsley

CONVENTIONAL (15 MINUTES)

1 HEAT the oil in the frypan, add the onions and mushrooms, and cook over medium heat for 3 minutes. Then add the tomatoes, eggs and parsley.
2 TURN the heat down to low, and cover the pan. Cook for 4 minutes.
3 ALLOW to stand for 4 minutes, then slice.

Serve the omelette with a green salad (page 86).

teaspoon
chopping board
knife
fork
non-stick frypan, and lid
egg lifter
knife (for slicing omelette)

MICROWAVE (7 MINUTES)

1 HEAT the oil in the microwave-safe container, uncovered, on HIGH (100%) for 30 seconds. Stir in the onions and mushrooms, and cook, uncovered, on HIGH (100%) for 2 minutes. Drain away any excess liquid.
2 ADD the tomatoes, eggs and parsley. Cover, and cook on HIGH (100%) for 3 minutes in the centre of the oven.
3 ALLOW to stand for 1 minute, then slice.

Serve the omelette with a green salad (page 86).

teaspoon
medium-sized microwave-safe container, and lid
chopping board
knife
fork
egg lifter
knife (for slicing omelette)

HANDY MAN HINTS

- *Mushrooms have a meaty flavour and are low in kilojoules. Add them to BBQs, dishes, salads, soups and casseroles.*
- *Try oyster mushrooms (page 67) for a lighter flavour.*

Manpower Milkshake

SERVES 1

2 cups low-fat milk
1 banana, roughly chopped
1 egg
50 g dried apricots, roughly chopped
1 tsp cinnamon

CONVENTIONAL (5 MINUTES)

1 PLACE all the ingredients in a blender.
2 BLEND for 2 minutes, shaking the jug halfway through this time.

Serve in a long glass.

cup measure
blender, or bowl and fork (see page 22)
knife
chopping board
teaspoon
long glass

HANDY MAN HINTS

- *Add 2 tablespoons of low-fat vanilla icecream to make this a high-energy snack.*
- *Bananas continue to ripen once picked; include some green ones when buying bananas and you will always have some ready to use.*

V8 Heart Starter

SERVES 1

250 ml V8 Juice
1 dash tabasco or Worcestershire sauce
ice cubes
1 slice lemon

CONVENTIONAL (2 MINUTES)

1 PLACE ice cubes in a long glass, and pour the juice over.
2 STIR in the sauce.

Serve with the slice of lemon.

can opener
glass
spoon

VARIATION *Substitute tomato juice for V8 juice.*

Mustard Scrambled Eggs in One

SERVES 1

2 tsp olive oil
2 (55 g) eggs, whisked
2 tbsp low-fat milk (80 ml)
1 tsp wholegrain mustard
1 tbsp fresh parsley, or ½ tsp dried
2 slices multigrain or wholemeal bread, toasted

CONVENTIONAL (5 MINUTES)

teaspoon
tablespoon
non-stick frypan
large breakfast bowl
fork
serving spoon

1 WHISK the eggs, milk, mustard and parsley together in a bowl with the fork.
2 HEAT the oil in a non-stick frypan over low heat, then add the egg mixture.
3 COOK over medium heat for 3–4 minutes, stirring continuously with the fork.

Serve on toast.

MICROWAVE (2½–3 MINUTES)

teaspoon
tablespoon
large breakfast bowl
tablespoon
fork
serving spoon

1 HEAT the oil in the bowl, uncovered, on HIGH (100%) for 30 seconds.
2 MIX in the eggs, milk, mustard and parsley, and beat with the fork for 30 seconds.
3 COOK, uncovered, on HIGH (100%) for 1½–2 minutes in 30-second bursts, stirring with the fork in between, until light and fluffy. Allow to stand for 1 minute to set the egg.

Serve on toast.

HANDY MAN HINTS

- *To whisk, use a fork.*
- *Eggs will cook more evenly if they are at room temperature.*

Toast Toppers

SERVES 1

140 g can baked beans
140 g can spaghetti
140 g can creamed corn
2 slices of wholegrain toast
1 tsp chopped parsley

CONVENTIONAL (5 MINUTES)

can opener
spoon
small saucepan
chopping board
knife

1 SPOON all the ingredients, except the toast, into the saucepan.
2 COOK according to the directions on the cans.
3 SPOON onto the toast.

Serve sprinkled with chopped parsley.

MICROWAVE (2 MINUTES)

can opener
spoon
small microwave-safe container, and lid
chopping board
knife

1 SPOON the ingredients into the microwave-safe container. Cover, and cook on HIGH (100%) for 1 minute.
2 SPOON onto the toast.

Serve sprinkled with chopped parsley.

FIT TIP *Look for no-added-salt varieties in cans.*

MIND POWER

'It's the mind that makes the body'

— Yoga slogan.

Our brains are 85% water, and if deprived of this fluid our thought processes and emotional stability are the first to dry up. So ensure you drink plenty of water — at least 6–8 glasses each day — and beat the afternoon 'office blues' with some energy-boosting foods.

FIT TIPS

- Our mouth is very close to our brain, yet we rarely think of food as having an impact on our ability to perform mentally. In fact, the foods we eat have a very important role to play in helping us concentrate and think clearly throughout the day. A high carbohydrate intake distributed at regular intervals over the day is the key to peak brain power.
- These carbo-loaded easy meal and snack ideas are perfect for the office, school, or out and about, and do not require a lot of brain power to prepare!

High-performance Snacks (page 33)

Sandwich Sensations (page 34)

Big Red Herbed Tomato Soup (page 58)

Pasta, Noodles or Rice (pages 111–13)

Mountain Bread with Chicken Curry and Corn (page 35)

Jaffle Jaz (page 36)

The Ace of Spuds (page 56)

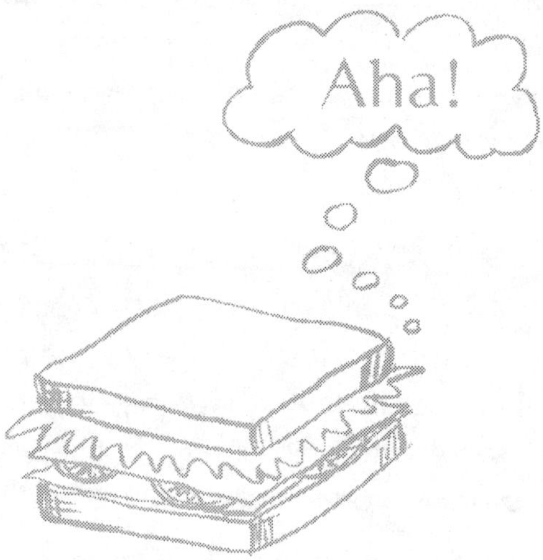

High-performance Snacks

- English multigrain muffins, toasted, with jam, honey, or golden syrup
- Low-fat fruit yoghurt
- Dried fruit: apricots, sultanas, raisins, figs, dates
- Low-fat fruit cake or fruit muffins
- Rice Cakes with honey and banana, or low-fat dip
- Wholemeal fruit bars (choose those with less than 10% fat)
- Muesli bars
- Low-fat pretzels
- Cup of soup (low-salt)
- Pancake with maple syrup
- Low-fat soft-serve icecream or yoghurt
- Crumpet with honey
- Fresh fruit salad
- Low-fat creamy rice
- Dry cereal (e.g. NutriGrain, MiniWheats, Wheat Bites, etc.).

Sandwich Sensations

Choose multigrain or wholemeal varieties of bread, or for a change, have a roll or bagel or pita bread. Omit the butter and margarine, and use instead a little ricotta cheese, light mayonnaise or a thin spread of avocado.

- Lean ham, pickles, tomato, and lettuce.
- Boiled egg mashed with mayo, and lettuce.
- Lean roast beef, mustard, grated carrot, and Swiss cheese.
- Sliced turkey, cranberry sauce, canned asparagus, and lettuce.
- Vegemite, low-fat cheddar cheese, and sprouts.
- Sliced meatloaf (page 101), chutney, and lettuce.
- Corned beef, pickles, and lettuce.
- Pork, apple sauce, currants, and cucumber slices.
- Leftover sausage or hamburger, sliced tomato and beetroot, with small lettuce leaves.
- Egg, wholegrain mustard, and lettuce.
- Sliced tomato, pickles, and lettuce.
- Capsicum, tomato, salami, and chilli sauce.
- Tuna, spring onions, and tomato.
- Lean chicken, and mango chutney.
- Baked beans and a dash of tabasco sauce.

HANDY MAN HINTS

- *To prevent soggy sandwiches, place the lettuce directly onto the bread slice.*
- *Sandwiches can be toasted, but let the toast go cold before wrapping. Toasting is particularly good for using up stale bread.*

Mountain Bread with Chicken and Corn

Serves 2

200 g skinless cooked chicken, shredded
160 g light cream cheese
1 lemon, juiced
1 (310 g) can sweetcorn kernels, drained
50 g alfalfa sprouts
2 slices mountain bread

scales
lemon juicer
bowl
spoon
plastic wrap
knife

CONVENTIONAL (5 MINUTES)

1 COMBINE half the chicken, cream cheese, lemon juice, corn and alfalfa sprouts in a bowl.
2 SPOON this mixture onto one side of the mountain bread, and roll up. Cover the roll with plastic wrap, twisting each end to keep the roll firm.
3 REPEAT the procedure with the remaining ingredients.

Refrigerate the rolls until you need them, then cut them in half, and serve.

HANDY MAN HINT *If you gradually unwrap the plastic as you eat, the roll will be easier to handle.*

VARIATIONS *Shredded ham, BBQ chicken or leftovers.*

Jaffle Jaz

Serves 2

4 slices wholemeal bread
20 g margarine or cooking oil spray
2 slices lean ham
½ tomato, sliced
1 (130 g) can baked beans

scales
chopping board
serrated knife
table knife
can opener
spoon

CONVENTIONAL (10 MINUTES)

Preheat the jaffle-maker.

1 SPREAD margarine on both sides of the bread slices, and place one slice of bread in each of the cavities.
2 COVER the bread with slices of ham and tomato, and the baked beans.
3 TOP with a slice of bread, and cook until the indicator lights up or until the jaffles are browned and crispy.

Serve immediately. Beware of the hot filling!

VARIATIONS *Other filling ideas:*

- *light cream cheese with chopped dried fruit*
- *peanut butter with banana*
- *grated carrot with peanut butter and sultanas (carrots can be purchased already grated)*
- *light cream cheese with tuna, capers and olives.*

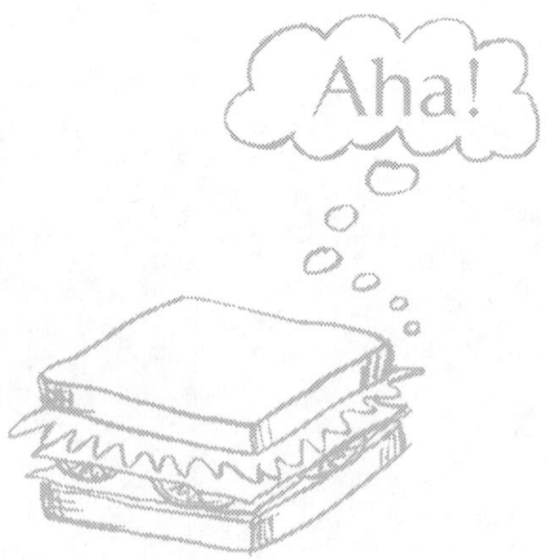

FOWL PLAY

'Give 'em curry, they need the runs'

— Aussie slogan at the Gabba,
Australia vs Pakistan match, 1996.

The most popular purchase from the supermarkets are BBQ chooks, as they make for the fast, freestyle meals, particularly after work or exercising. Combined with a can from the shelf, a few fresh ingredients, and with the skin and fat removed chicken is fit, fast and filling food.

Current research from supermarkets indicates that they do not regard each other as their main competitors, but rather fast food chains where young people and double-income families eat a large proportion of their meals. This has contributed to us being officially the second-most obese race after the citizens of the USA — not a good look, or a good prognosis for a long and healthy life!

FIT TIP

- Chicken is a good source of protein and many B vitamins. However it can also be high in fat and cholesterol. Fix this quickly in one 'fowl' swoop by removing the skin. Just remember that it is only when it is cooked that the skin looks appealing, so remove it before you cook, and you will not even be tempted!

Dinner in a Dash, with a BBQ Chook

Chicken and Pasta Salad

Add a can of chopped tomatoes, and some olives, to cooked pasta, and toss through strips of BBQ chicken.

Chicken and Warm Potato Salad

Replace the sausage in Peak-hour Potato and Sausage-sizzle Salad (page 83) with chicken strips.

Chicken Noodles

Mix together a can of whole baby corn, a handful of snowpeas, and hot cooked noodles, and toss with strips of BBQ chicken, a splash of soy sauce, a squeeze of lime juice and a dash of sweet chilli sauce.

Chicken Roll

Wrap a mixture of shredded BBQ chicken, salad and a dip sauce in mountain bread.

Chicken and Rice

Stir shredded BBQ chicken through hot cooked rice, and add some shredded raw carrot, and peas. Toss with BBQ sauce.

Nasi Goreng

Add a can of prawns, some cooked peas and rice seasonings to hot cooked white rice. Toss with diced BBQ chicken and a splash of soy sauce. Top with unsalted peanuts.

Soul Men

Satay Chicken in the Bag (page 42)
Cucumber Raita Salad (page 78)
Hokkein Noodles (page 43)

If you've had an active day, make the serve of noodles a big one! Finish with some fresh fruit to get your fill of antioxidants and carbohydrate.

Stirring Stuff

Howzat? — Honey-chicken stir-fry (page 44)
Steamed Rice (pages 112, 113)
Green with Envy Salad (page 86)
Flash Fruit Salad (page 168)

Stir-frying is a great way of cooking vegetables to retain maximum nutrition. Your vegetables should be crisp and crunchy in a stir-fry, not limp and floppy! The brighter their colour, the more vitamins they have retained.

Heart Starter

Ten-minute Thai Curry (page 45)
Steamed Rice (pages 112, 113)
Lychees and melon wedges (page 193)

This superb curry will not only start your heart but as it is low in fat it will help keep your heart healthy for a long time.

Championship Chook

Chicken Balls with Gnocchi and Tomato (page 46)
Fresh berries, with Vitari ice confection (available in freezers at supermarkets)

Pasta is a great source of carbohydrate for lasting energy; however, it is important to choose low-fat sauces to accompany it. Tomato-based sauces are usually a good choice.

You may wish to include some lean chicken, beef or seafood for protein, but avoid salami and other high-fat processed meats.

Chicken Zip

Mexican Chick (page 47)
Some-like-it-hot Mexican Rice (page 48)
Honeyed Carrot Salad (page 81)

Mexican food available in Australia is typically very high in fat, with sour cream, cheese and avocado featuring heavily. However, the seasoning, beans and rice components of Mexican cooking are very healthy, and can form the basis of some very tasty dishes.

How to Roast Chicken

SERVES 2–4

1 large onion, peeled and cut in half
size 12 chicken (1.2 kg), thawed
½ tsp dried mixed herbs
15 g margarine, melted
black pepper, freshly ground, to taste
1 tbsp sweet paprika (microwave method only)

CONVENTIONAL (50 MINUTES)

Preheat the oven to 180°C.

1 WASH the chicken, and dry it thoroughly. Pierce the skin in three places with a fork or skewer. Place half the onion in the cavity. Roughly chop the other half onion, and combine it with the herbs and the melted margarine.

2 PLACE the chicken on the baking tray, and brush the chicken with the herb 'butter'. Bake in the middle of the oven for 45 minutes, turning the chicken over halfway through the cooking time.

Allow to stand for 5 minutes, then remove the skin before cutting and serving.

chopping board
knife
teaspoon
scales
tablespoon
fork
metal baking tray
pastry brush
carving dish
carving knife and fork

MICROWAVE (30 MINUTES)

1 WASH the chicken, and dry it thoroughly. Pierce the skin in three places with a fork or a skewer. Place half the onion in the cavity. Roughly chop the other half onion, and combine it with the herbs and the melted margarine.

2 PLACE the chicken on the microwave-safe roasting rack, brush the chicken with the herb butter, and sprinkle with paprika.

3 COVER loosely with paper towel, and cook on HIGH (100%) for 24 minutes, turning the chicken over halfway through the cooking time.

Allow to stand for 5 minutes, then remove the skin before cutting and serving.

chopping board
knife
teaspoon
scales
tablespoon
fork
microwave-safe roasting rack
pastry brush
non-recycled paper towel
carving dish
carving knife and fork

VARIATION *For garlic flavour, bake a whole unpeeled garlic bulb beside the chicken. For low-fat chicken, remove the skin, and cook the chicken in an oven bag. The bonus — no messy oven to clean!*

Satay Chicken, in the Bag

SERVES 2

2 chicken skinless fillets, sliced into strips
1 pkt of mild Satay Shakers

Satay dipping sauce
½ cup peanut butter
¾ cup water
1 tbsp tomato paste
1 tbsp salt-reduced soy sauce

CONVENTIONAL (25 MINUTES)

Preheat the oven to 180°C.

1 PLACE the chicken strips inside the plastic bag, add the contents of the chicken shaker, and shake until all the chicken strips are evenly coated.
2 PLACE the chicken strips on a tray lined with baking paper, and bake in the oven for 15–20 minutes until they are browned.
3 TO MAKE the satay sauce: Place all the sauce ingredients in a bowl, and mix together thoroughly.

Serve with the satay dipping sauce, and rice (pages 113, 114).

chopping board
knife
plastic bag
cup measure
tablespoon
metal baking tray
baking paper
mixing bowl
serving spoon

MICROWAVE (5 MINUTES)

1 COMBINE all the ingredients in the microwave-safe container.
2 COVER, and cook on HIGH (100%) for 2–3 minutes.
3 STIR, and allow to stand for 1 minute, covered loosely with paper towel.

Serve with rice (pages 113, 114).

chopping board
knife
cup measure
tablespoon
medium-sized microwave-safe container, and lid
non-recycled paper towel
serving spoon

HANDY MAN HINT

If you use baking paper, you will save on the washing up.

Hokkien Noodles

SERVES 2

2 tsp sesame oil
1 red pepper, sliced
200 g fresh oyster mushrooms, sliced
6 spring onions, chopped
2 small red chillies, seeded and chopped
1 pkt fresh egg noodles
⅓ cup Ketjap Manis Indonesian Sweet Soya Sauce

teaspoon
chopping board
knife
wok or non-stick frypan
wooden spoon
bowl
serving spoon

CONVENTIONAL (5 MINUTES)

1 HEAT the oil in a wok or frypan over high heat for 30 seconds. Add the pepper and mushrooms and cook for 2 minutes, stirring occasionally, until the pepper is soft.
2 ADD the onions and chillies, and cook for 2 minutes, until the onions are soft.
3 TOSS the noodles and the soy sauce in a bowl and stir into the mixture. Cook over medium heat for 2 minutes until the noodles are hot.

Serve immediately.

HANDY MAN HINT

Like pasta and rice, these noodles reheat quickly in a microwave oven. Place 4 cups noodles in a bowl; then cover, and cook on HIGH (100%) for 2 minutes.

Howzat? — Honey-chicken Stir-fry

Serves 2

1 tbsp olive oil
1 onion, chopped
100 g mushrooms, sliced
300 g lean skinless chicken, thinly sliced
75 g snowpeas, topped and tailed
2 tbsp honey and 2 tbsp soy sauce, combined

CONVENTIONAL (10 MINUTES)

tablespoon
chopping board
knife
small bowl
spoon
non-stick frypan or wok
wooden spoon
serving spoon

1 HEAT the oil in the frypan over medium heat, and stir-fry the onion and mushrooms over medium heat for 2 minutes.
2 ADD the remaining ingredients, and stir through evenly.
3 COOK over high heat for 5 minutes, stirring frequently.

Serve over steamed rice (pages 113, 114).

MICROWAVE (10 MINUTES)

tablespoon
chopping board
knife
large microwave-safe container, and lid
serving spoon

1 COMBINE the oil, onion and mushrooms in the microwave-safe container. Cook, uncovered, on HIGH (100%) for 2 minutes.
2 STIR, then add the remaining ingredients, and stir through evenly.
3 COOK, uncovered, on HIGH (100%) for 5 minutes, stirring halfway through the cooking time.

Serve over steamed rice (pages 113, 114).

HANDY MAN HINTS

- *To make bottled honey runny: remove the metal lid from the jar first, then heat the jar in the microwave oven on HIGH (100%) for ½–1 minute.*
- *Honey is a natural antiseptic and antibiotic, and has been used in mainstream medicine to treat conditions such as tonsillitis and stomach ulcers.*

Ten-minute Thai Curry

SERVES 2

1 tbsp olive oil
1 onion, diced
2 tsp green curry paste
200 g pumpkin, peeled and cut into 2 cm cubes
300 g skinless chicken fillets, sliced thinly
100 g frozen beans
1 (140 g) can low-fat coconut milk

CONVENTIONAL (25 MINUTES)

tablespoon
chopping board
knife
teaspoon
scales
can opener
non-stick frypan
wooden spoon
serving spoon

1 HEAT the oil in the frypan over medium heat for 30 seconds. Then add the onion and curry paste, and cook for 2 minutes.
2 STIR in the pumpkin, chicken, beans and coconut milk, and simmer over medium heat for 15 minutes, stirring twice, until the chicken is tender.
3 ALLOW to stand for 3 minutes.

Serve with rice (pages 113, 114).

MICROWAVE (9–12 MINUTES)

tablespoon
chopping board
knife
teaspoon
scales
can opener
large microwave-safe container, and lid
serving spoon

1 PLACE the oil, onion and curry paste in the microwave-safe container. Cover, and cook on HIGH (100%) for 2 minutes.
2 ADD the pumpkin, chicken, beans and coconut milk. Cover, and cook on HIGH (100%) for 3–4 minutes, stirring halfway through the cooking time.
3 STIR, and allow to stand for 4 minutes.

Serve with rice (pages 113, 114).

HANDY MAN HINT

Add 1 tbsp chopped fresh coriander or mint leaves to the curry, and garnish with 2 tbsp unsalted peanuts.

Chicken Balls with Gnocchi and Tomato

SERVES 2

200 g lean chicken mince
2 tbsp breadcrumbs
1 tbsp plum sauce
1 tsp dried basil (or 1 tbsp fresh basil, chopped)
1 (55 g) egg
½ cup flour
1 (370 g) jar Italian-style tomato pasta sauce
1 (625 g) pkt gnocchi (cooked)

CONVENTIONAL (15–20 MINUTES)

1 COMBINE all the ingredients, except the pasta sauce, in a food processor and blend until smooth.
2 PLACE 1 sheet of foil on the bench and sprinkle it with the flour. Roll the meat mixture in the flour, and shape into 10 walnut-sized balls.
3 PLACE in the frypan, and cook over medium heat for 6–8 minutes stirring three times during the cooking.
4 ADD the pasta sauce, and cook, uncovered, to heat through for 5 minutes.

Serve over the cooked gnocchi.

chopping board
knife
tablespoon
teaspoon
cup measure
can opener
spoon
food processor, or bowl and fork
foil
non-stick frypan
wooden spoon

MICROWAVE (8–10 MINUTES)

1 COMBINE all the ingredients, except the pasta sauce, in a food processor and blend until smooth.
2 PLACE 1 sheet of foil on the bench and sprinkle it with the flour. Roll the meat mixture in the flour, and shape it into 10 walnut-sized balls.
3 PLACE the chicken balls in the microwave-safe container. Cook, uncovered, on HIGH (100%) for 2 minutes.
4 ADD the pasta sauce. Cover, and cook on HIGH (100%) for 3–4 minutes to heat through.

Serve over the cooked gnocchi.

chopping board
knife
tablespoon
teaspoon
cup measure
can opener
spoon
food processor, or bowl and fork
foil
medium-sized microwave-safe container, and lid

HANDY MAN HINT

Chicken cooked in the microwave is excellent if you are 'waist watching', as you can eliminate the fat, and the cooked result is speedy and tender.

Mexican Chick

SERVES 2

2 skinless chicken breasts (300 g), of even thickness
1 tbsp lemon juice
1 tbsp olive oil
1 tbsp tomato paste
1 tsp Mexican seasoning

CONVENTIONAL (1 HOUR; 10 MINUTES)

tablespoon
teaspoon
shallow dish or container
spoon
non-stick frypan
slotted spoon

1 COMBINE all the ingredients in a shallow container, and leave to marinate for 1 hour, if possible.
2 HEAT the frypan over low heat, remove the chicken breasts from the marinade and cook them for 6–8 minutes, turning them over halfway through the cooking time.
3 ALLOW to stand for 1 minute.

Serve with Mexican Salsa (page 153).

MICROWAVE (1 HOUR; 6 MINUTES)

tablespoon
teaspoon
shallow microwave-safe container
spoon
non-recycled paper towel

1 COMBINE all the ingredients in the microwave-safe container, and leave to marinate for 1 hour if possible.
2 COVER the container loosely with paper towel, and cook on HIGH (100%) for 5 minutes, turning the chicken breasts halfway through the cooking time.
3 ALLOW the chicken to stand for 1 minute.

Serve with Mexican Salsa (page 153).

HANDY MAN HINT *Pound the chicken fillets into even thickness with a meat mallet to ensure that they cook evenly and quickly.*

VARIATION *Shred the chicken, and add to rice or pasta.*

Some-like-it-hot Mexican Rice

SERVES 2

1 (270 g) can sweetcorn kernels
100 g frozen green beans
3 spring onions, chopped
2 tsp Mexican spice
2½ cups cooked rice (pages 113, 114), at room temperature

CONVENTIONAL (8–10 MINUTES)

can opener
chopping board
knife
teaspoon
cup measure
non-stick frypan
wooden spoon

1 HEAT the frypan, and add the corn, beans, onions and spice, mixing through evenly.
2 COOK over medium heat for 5 minutes, stirring constantly.
3 STIR in the rice, and mix together. Cook the rice mixture over medium heat for a further 3 minutes to heat through.

Serve with taco sauce, or Jalapeno cheese sauce, or your favourite sauce.

MICROWAVE (6–8 MINUTES)

can opener
chopping board
knife
teaspoon
cup measure
medium-sized microwave-safe container, and lid
spoon

1 COMBINE the corn, beans, onions, and spice in the microwave-safe container, mixing through evenly. Cover, and cook on HIGH (100%) for 4 minutes, stirring halfway through the cooking time.
2 ADD the rice, and mix through evenly. Cover and cook on HIGH (100%) for 2 minutes.

Serve with taco sauce, or Jalapeno cheese sauce, or your favourite sauce.

HANDY MAN HINT *Freeze leftovers to defrost for a snack down the track. Otherwise take the leftovers to work for a carbohydrate boost during the day.*

FIT TIP *It is time to rehabilitate starch, as it is filling without being fattening, and helps prevent colon cancer.*

VEGING OUT

'Large, naked raw carrots are acceptable as food only to those who live in hutches eagerly awaiting Easter'

— Fran Lebowitz.

Vegetables do not feature high up on most Australians' shopping list, and I suspect that meat and three veg, steak and frozen chips, sausages and mash, are more often than not served at home. There are many horror stories about vegetables from people who have suffered badly cooked vegetables from the hands of old-fashioned cooks (could this be Mum?). They cite cabbage, Brussel sprouts and broccoli as their turnoffs from venturing far from chips, peas and tomatoes.

Vegies are on the decline: We know that vegetables are good for us, but we are eating less now than at any time in the past nine years, according to the Australian Bureau of Statistics. We have even cooled towards spuds — consumption of this favourite is down by 7.1 per cent.

Our diversity of produce is second to none, and, believe me, it's cheap to boot, by world standards.

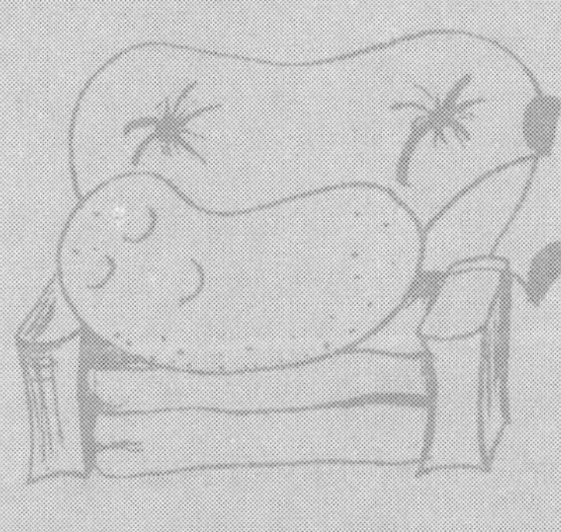

Australia's favourite groceries

The top ten products each had sales in Australia of more than $110 million last year:

1 Coca Cola
2 Nescafé instant coffee
3 Pedigree Pal dog food
4 Kraft cheeses
5 Tip Top bread
6 Sorbent toilet paper
7 Buttercup bread
8 Huggies nappies
9 Whiskas cat food
10 Cadbury block chocolate

(*Age*, 4 February 1997)

Fit tips

- Everybody knows that vegetables are good for them, but sometimes finding quick and interesting ways to prepare them just gets a little too difficult.
- Keep in mind that frozen and canned vegetables are a nutritious and convenient alternative to fresh vegetables. Even if you are organised enough to shop regularly for fresh vegetables, always keep some frozen ones on hand for the times when you run out.
- Aim to eat at least five serves of vegetables each day, which is not difficult if you consider the following menus.

Couch Potatoes

Macho Minestrone — Soup with the Lot (page 55)
The Ace of Spuds (page 56)

A great TV dinner after a hard day at work, this meal will not only fill your stomach but ensure full muscle glycogen stores (the muscles' most important energy store, made from carbohydrate).

Winter Warmer

Big Red Herbed Tomato Soup (page 58)
Fit Fritters (page 59)
Mountains of Mash (page 60)

In cold weather we look for comfort food, much of it is high in fat. Most can be made low-fat very simply — by using fat-reduced ingredients, and preparing them with a minimum of oil, butter or cream. This menu will defrost an Eskimo, and keep him lean as a bonus!

Peak-hour Potatoes and Pizza

The Big Easy — Potato and Corn Chowder (page 61)
Pizza Mushrooms (page 62)
Low-fat icecream and fruit (pages 190, 191)

A thick soup can be a meal in itself, particularly if it includes potato or grains, a little meat or chicken, and plenty of vegetables. If you have a lot of meals without meat, mushrooms are a good food to eat regularly, as they are the only plant source of vitamin B_{12}.

Easy on the Eyes

Pumpkin Soup for Punters (page 63)
Easy Vegetable Lasagne (page 64)

Vegetables with a deep orange or red colour are a good source of carotene or vitamin A, which is not only essential for seeing in the dark but is believed to be an important antioxidant. This meal is loaded with vitamin A and many other essential vitamins, not to mention dietary fibre and carbohydrate galore.

Real Men Do Eat Vegetables

Big-flavour Bubble 'n' Squeak (page 65)
Cauliflower Cheese Knockout (page 66)

Here are a couple of old favourites that make eating vegies easy. If you squash the vegies or hide them with a sauce, they taste too good to be good for you! Cheese sauce (the low-fat way) boosts your calcium intake if you don't drink a lot of milk!

How to Cook Vegetables

A general rule is to start cooking vegetables that grow underground (root vegetables) in cold water; those that grow above the ground in boiling water (use a minimum of water — steaming is better), which brings out the chlorophyll or green colour. Do not overcook green vegetables or they will lose their colour and vitamins, so stop cooking when they are just tender, and then drain them immediately.

How to Microwave Vegetables

To retain more nutrients than you can with traditionally boiled vegetables:

- Chop vegies into equal sizes of about 3 cm.
- Rinse the vegetables well, and do not add excess water so that they cook quickly and retain their colour and flavour.
- Do not add salt, as it will dry out the vegies. Only season at the table, if it is really desired.
- Use microwave-safe cookware and cover to cook.
- Cook the vegetables on HIGH (100%); the timing depends on the type of vegetable and the number of pieces.

Here's a rule of thumb:

- hard-fibred vegetables (e.g. potatoes, carrots, corn) — per 500 g, cook on HIGH (100%) for 6–8 minutes
- soft-fibred vegetables (e.g. asparagus, tomatoes, zucchini) — per 500 g, cook on HIGH (100%) for 4–6 minutes.

For the bone lazy, it is better to leave the skin on the vegetables to maintain the maximum vitamin and fibre content.

FIT TIP *Freshly frozen vegetables are often nutritionally equivalent to fresh vegies, and are convenient for lazy shoppers!*

How to Barbecue Vegetables

Serves 2

3 large washed potatoes, sliced into ½ cm rounds (include sweet potato if desired)
250 g button mushrooms, brushed with a little olive oil
1 onion, peeled and sliced into rings
2 medium-sized tomatoes, halved

chopping board
knife
pastry brush
egg lifter or tongs

Conventional (20 minutes)

1 BRUSH the preheated barbecue plate with oil. Place the potatoes on the plate, and cook for 15 minutes, turning halfway through the cooking time.
2 ADD the onions, mushrooms and tomatoes, and cook for a further 10 minutes, turning the vegetables halfway through the cooking time.

Serve with Lemony Lamb Racks (page 94).

Handy Man Hints *To speed the cooking of potatoes, zap them in a microwave oven for 2 minutes before barbecuing. Or place the potatoes in a large saucepan, cover with water and bring to the boil; drain and allow to cool slightly.*

Variation *Use sweet potatoes in place of potatoes.*

BBQ Corn on the Cob

4 corn cobs, fresh or frozen
black pepper, freshly ground, to taste

Serves 2

CONVENTIONAL (8 MINUTES)

chopping board
tongs

1 PULL the husk off, and remove the silk threads. Rinse, and season the cobs.
2 PREHEAT BBQ and place the cobs on the metal plate of a preheated barbecue.
3 COOK for 5–6 minutes, turning the cobs over at 2-minute intervals.

Serve immediately.

MICROWAVE (5 MINUTES EACH COB)

chopping board
tongs

1 PULL the husk off each cob and remove the silk threads. Rinse and season the cobs.
2 COVER again with the husks, and cook 1 cob on HIGH (100%) for 3 minutes, turning the cob halfway through the cooking time. Remove the husk. Repeat for the other cobs.

Serve immediately.

HANDY MAN HINTS

- *More food takes more time to cook in a microwave oven. Cook 4 cobs on HIGH (100%) for 9 minutes.*
- *Rub the corn cobs before cooking with freshly crushed garlic.*

Minestrone Macho — Soup with the Lot

SERVES 2

1 tbsp olive oil
1 onion, finely diced
2 rashers rindless lean bacon, cut into strips
1 cup frozen mixed vegetables
1 (425 g) can tomato soup
2 tbsp grated Parmesan cheese

CONVENTIONAL (10 MINUTES)

1 COMBINE the oil, onion and bacon in the saucepan, and brown over low heat for 2 minutes, stirring occasionally
2 STIR in the vegetables and soup. Cover, and cook over low heat for 6–8 minutes.
3 STIR the soup well, then pour into bowls. Sprinkle with cheese.

Serve with crusty bread.

tablespoon
chopping board
cup measure
can opener
large saucepan, and lid
wooden spoon
serving bowls

MICROWAVE (8–10 MINUTES)

1 COMBINE the oil, onion and bacon in the microwave-safe container. Cook, uncovered, on HIGH (100%) for 1½ minutes.
2 STIR in the vegetables and soup. Cover, and cook on HIGH (100%) for 5 minutes until the soup boils. Allow to stand for 1 minute.
3. STIR the soup well, then pour into bowl. Sprinkle with cheese.

Serve with crusty bread.

tablespoon
chopping board
cup measure
can opener
large microwave-safe container, and lid
spoon
serving bowls

VARIATIONS
- *Stir in 1 cup cooked pasta or rice for a really hearty meal.*
- *Add 1 small can baked beans at step 2.*

The Ace of Spuds — Jacket Potatoes, a Meal in One

Serves 2

4 medium-sized potatoes (700 g), washed and pierced four times with a fork;
topping of your choice (see page 57)

CONVENTIONAL (1 HOUR)

fork
chopping board
knife

Preheat the oven to 200°C.

1 PLACE the prepared potatoes on a rack in the middle of the oven and bake for 45 minutes–1 hour, until cooked through. Allow to stand until the potatoes are cool enough to handle.
2 CUT the potatoes in half, add your favourite topping: grated cheese, a sprinkle of paprika or chopped parsley, etc.

MICROWAVE (10 MINUTES)

fork
chopping board
knife

1 PLACE the prepared potatoes on the edge of the turntable.
2 COOK, uncovered, on HIGH (100%) for 8 minutes, turning the potatoes over halfway through the cooking time.
3 ALLOW to stand until the potatoes are cool enough to handle. Cut the potatoes in half, and add your preferred topping: grated cheese, a sprinkle of paprika or chopped parsley, etc.

HANDY MAN HINTS

- *When buying potatoes, choose potatoes free from sprouts and greenish tinges.*
- *Buy loose potatoes, not those in plastic bags, but if you do buy them in plastic remove the plastic before storing.*
- *Store in a cool, dry, dark place, never in the fridge. Warmth can cause sprouting, damp can cause rot, and light can cause greening (which is poisonous).*
- *Cover baked potatoes loosely with non-recycled paper towel, and reheat in the microwave oven on HIGH (100%) for 1½–2 minutes.*

Top Ten Potato Toppers

An average potato contains about 367 Kj, and is virtually fat free. It's the topping you need to watch!

1 Combine light sour cream and chopped chives.
2 Three-bean mix, with a dash of Mexican spice — wind-powered potatoes!
3 Choice of three cheeses: blue, fetta, mozzarella.
4 Combine shredded BBQ chicken and mayo.
5 Combine cooked lean bacon and light sour cream.
6 Steamed herbed mushrooms.
7 Coleslaw (see page 79).
8 Your favourite bottled pesto.
9 Steamed asparagus and ham, with light sour cream.
10 Roast beef, thinly sliced, with sour cream and horseradish.

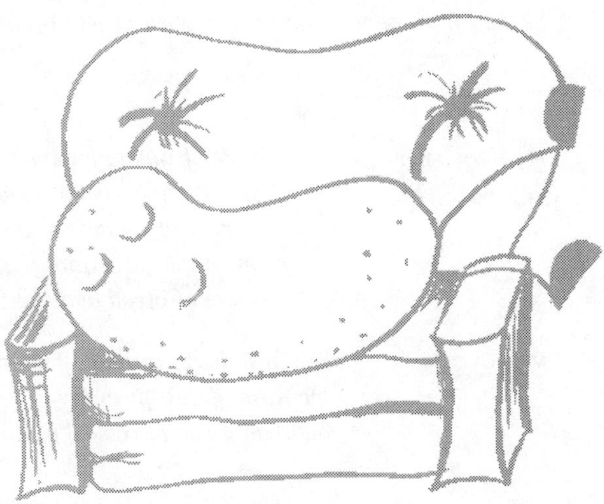

Big Red Herbed Tomato Soup

SERVES 2

1 (425 g) can tomato soup
1 soup can low-fat milk
1 tsp dried mixed herbs
dash of tabasco sauce (optional)
1 tbsp chopped fresh mixed herbs
black pepper, freshly ground, to taste
crusty bread

CONVENTIONAL (12 MINUTES)

can opener
wooden spoon
large saucepan
teaspoon
chopping board
knife
tablespoon

1 COMBINE the soup, milk and herbs in the saucepan, stirring well, and reheat over medium heat for 5–10 minutes, stirring several times so that it does not boil.

Season with pepper, and serve with crusty bread.

MICROWAVE (8 MINUTES)

can opener
wooden spoon
large microwave-safe container, and lid
chopping board
knife
tablespoon

1 COMBINE the soup and herbs in the microwave-safe container. Cover, and cook on HIGH (100%) for 2 minutes.

2 STIR in the milk. Cover, and cook on HIGH (100%) for 3–4 minutes. Do not boil.

Season with pepper, and serve with crusty bread.

HANDY MAN HINTS

- *Rule of thumb for tabasco sauce: ¼ tsp tabasco sauce is equal to ½ tsp ground black pepper, ½ tsp white pepper or a pinch of cayene pepper.*
- *In winter a thermos flask of soup is filling with a piece of bread and some fresh fruit.*

VARIATIONS

- *Use fresh herbs instead of dried to obtain a fresher flavour in the ratio of 1:3 (fresh:dry).*
- *Add half a cup of cooked pasta or rice for a heartier soup.*

Fit Fritters

SERVES 2

1 medium-sized zucchini, grated
1 (310 g) sweetcorn kernels, drained
1 sachet of the 'cup of soup' of your choice
2 (55 g) eggs
2 tbsp plain flour
1 tsp oil or cooking spray

CONVENTIONAL (10 MINUTES)

chopping board
grater
can opener
tablespoon
bowl
spoon
large non-stick frypan

1. COMBINE all the ingredients, except the oil and tomato sauce, together in the bowl, mixing evenly.
2. COVER the base of the frypan with the oil or cooking spray, and warm over medium heat for 1 minute.
3. PLACE level tablespoons of the mixture in the pan, and cook over medium heat for 5 minutes, turning them over halfway through the cooking time. Drain on paper towel, and put aside on a warmed plate. Repeat until all the mixture is used.

Serve with tomato sauce, chutney or pickles.

HANDY MAN HINT

Microwave corn on the cob for a quick low-fat snack. If the leaves have already been removed, wrap the cobs individually in plastic wrap; if the leaves are still on the cobs, cook them as they are. For one cob, cook on HIGH (100%) for 3–4 minutes.

VARIATIONS

Add any of the following: finely chopped onion, peppers, grated cheese or carrot, and herbs.

Mountains of Mash

Serves 2

4 large Desiree or pink potatoes (820 g), pierced six times with a fork
cold water to cover
2 tbsp low-fat milk
1½ tbsp margarine
salt and pepper, to taste

CONVENTIONAL (35 MINUTES)

fork
large saucepan, and lid
knife
tablespoon
potato masher

1 PLACE the prepared potatoes in a saucepan, and cover with the cold water. Cover, and bring to the boil. Reduce the heat, and simmer over low heat for 30 minutes, until fork tender.
2 ALLOW the potatoes to cool until you can handle them safely, then peel the potatoes.
3 Return the potatoes to the pan, add the milk, and mash with the fork or potato masher. Place the margarine on top of the mash, and beat until the margarine has melted and the potatoes are creamy.

Season to taste, and serve with Steak My Way (page 98).

MICROWAVE (15 MINUTES)

fork
medium-sized microwave-safe container
knife
tablespoon
potato masher

1 PLACE the prepared potatoes around the edge of the turntable, and cook, uncovered, on HIGH (100%) for 10 minutes.
2 ALLOW to stand until the potatoes are cool enough to handle, then peel the potatoes.
3 Place the potatoes in the microwave-safe container, add the milk, and mash with the fork or potato masher. Place the margarine on top of the mash. Cover, and cook on HIGH (100%) for 2 minutes, stirring once during the cooking time.
4 MIX the mash until it is creamy.

Season to taste, and serve with Steak My Way (page 98).

HANDY MAN HINTS

- *When buying your potatoes, choose a uniform size for even cooking, cook whole, then cut to size.*
- *New potatoes are best for boiling.*
- *Pink-skinned potatoes can add a touch of difference if left in their jackets.*

The Big Easy — Potato and Corn Chowder

SERVES 2

3 rashers rindless lean bacon, diced finely
4 spring onions, chopped
5 medium potatoes (900 g), peeled and cut into 2 cm cubes
2 tbsp water (microwave method only)
1 (270 g) can creamed corn
1 cup low-fat milk, mixed with 1 cup hot water
salt and pepper to taste

CONVENTIONAL (30 MINUTES)

chopping board
knife
potato peeler
can opener
cup measure
large saucepan
spoon

1 COOK the bacon and onion in a large saucepan over high heat for 2 minutes, stirring occasionally.
2 ADD the potatoes. Cover, and simmer over medium heat for 20 minutes, stirring three times during the cooking time.
3 ADD the corn, and milk and water. Cover, and cook over medium heat (do not boil), for a further 5 minutes stirring three times during the cooking time.

Season to taste, and serve with crusty bread.

MICROWAVE (25 MINUTES)

chopping board
knife
potato peeler
can opener
large microwave-safe container, and lid
can opener
cup measure
spoon

1 PLACE the bacon and onion in the microwave-safe container. Cook, uncovered, on HIGH (100%) for 1 minute.
2 ADD the potatoes and 2 tbsp water. Cover, and cook on HIGH (100%) for 10 minutes.
3 ADD the corn, and milk and water. Cover, and cook on HIGH (100%) for 10 minutes, stirring halfway through the cooking time.

Season to taste, and serve with crusty bread.

VARIATION *Stir a can of drained clams through the soup 3 minutes before the end of the cooking time for a version of American clam chowder.*

Pizza Mushrooms

SERVES 2

8 field-style mushrooms, stalks removed
8 tbsp pasta sauce
2 tsp chopped parsley
4 tbsp grated light mozzarella cheese

CONVENTIONAL (8 MINUTES)

chopping board
knife
tablespoon
teaspoon
foil
grill tray

1 PLACE 1 tbsp pasta sauce in each upturned mushroom cap, sprinkle with parsley, and top with cheese.
2 PLACE the mushrooms, gill side up, on a foil-lined grill tray.
3 COOK under a preheated, medium grill for 3–5 minutes, until the cheese is brown and bubbly.

Serve immediately.

MICROWAVE (5 MINUTES)

chopping board
knife
tablespoon
teaspoon
plain microwave-safe dinner plate
fork

1 PLACE 1 tbsp pasta sauce in each upturned mushroom cap, sprinkle with parsley, and top with cheese.
2 PLACE the mushrooms, gill side up, on the dinner plate in a circular pattern.
3 COOK, uncovered, on HIGH (100%) for 2–3 minutes, until the mushrooms are tender when tested with a fork.

Serve immediately.

VARIATION *Use shredded chicken, or ham with cheese, for the stuffing.*

Pumpkin Soup for Punters

SERVES 2

1 small butternut pumpkin (500 g)
2 cups vegetable stock, hot
2 spring onions, finely chopped
1 tbsp chopped chives
2 tsp nutmeg
½ cup low-fat milk

CONVENTIONAL (25 MINUTES)

1 PEEL and cube the pumpkin and place in the saucepan. Add the stock, cover, and simmer over medium heat for 15 minutes, or until the pumpkin is soft.
2 COOL the soup, and place it in a blender. Blend for 1–2 minutes, before returning to the saucepan with the onions, chives and nutmeg.
3 REHEAT the soup over medium heat, then stir in the milk to warm through, but do not boil.

Serve with crusty bread.

chopping board
knife
potato or pumpkin peeler
cup measure
tablespoon
teaspoon
blender or fork
large saucepan, and lid
wooden spoon
soup ladle

MICROWAVE (15 MINUTES)

1 PIERCE the unpeeled pumpkin six times with a fork, and place on an upturned microwave-safe plate. Cook on HIGH (100%) for 10–12 minutes. Allow to stand for 5 minutes.
2 WHEN it is cool enough to handle, cut the pumpkin in half lengthwise, and scoop out the flesh into a large microwave-safe bowl. Add the stock, onions, chives and nutmeg, and stir well.
3 COVER, and cook on HIGH (100%) for 4 minutes, stirring halfway through the cooking time. Stir in the milk.

Serve with crusty bread.

fork
microwave-safe plate
chopping board
knife
spoon
large microwave-safe bowl, and lid
cup measure
tablespoon
teaspoon
soup ladle

VARIATIONS

- *Add curry powder instead of the nutmeg.*
- *Add ½ cup sweetcorn kernels or canned prawns or 1 tbsp mixed fresh herbs, chopped.*
- *Replace the milk/cream with 1 tbsp natural yoghurt.*

Easy Vegetable Lasagne

Serves 4

2 cups (500 ml) pasta sauce
1 (200 g) eggplant, cut into 2 cm cubes
1 small green pepper, cut into 1 cm dice
8 instant lasagne sheets (100 g)
2 cups ricotta cheese
¼ cup grated light mozzarella cheese

CONVENTIONAL (1¼ HOURS)

cup measure
chopping board
knife
large saucepan, and lid
skewer
casserole dish
spoon

Preheat the oven to 190°C.

1 PLACE the pasta sauce, eggplant and pepper in the saucepan. Cover, and cook over medium heat for 15 minutes until the vegetables are skewer-soft.
2 ASSEMBLE the lasagne by spreading one-third of the pasta sauce over the base of the casserole dish. Cover this with four lasagne sheets, and then top it with one-third of the ricotta cheese. Repeat the procedure, finishing with a layer of ricotta cheese.
3 SPRINKLE the top of the lasagne with mozzarella cheese, and bake in the oven on the middle shelf for 45–50 minutes.

Allow to stand for 5 minutes before serving with a tossed green salad.

MICROWAVE (40 MINUTES)

cup measure
chopping board
knife
microwave-safe glass jug
plastic wrap
spoon
microwave-safe casserole dish

1 PLACE the pasta sauce, eggplant and pepper in a microwave-safe glass jug. Cover, and cook on HIGH (100%) for 10 minutes.
2 ASSEMBLE the lasagne by spreading one-third of the pasta sauce over the base of the microwave-safe casserole dish. Cover this with four lasagne sheets, and then top it with one-third of the ricotta cheese. Repeat the procedure, finishing with a layer of ricotta cheese.
3 SPRINKLE the top of the lasagne with mozzarella cheese. Cover with plastic wrap, and cook on MEDIUM (50–60%) for 25 minutes.

Allow to stand for 5 minutes before serving with a tossed green salad.

HANDY MAN HINTS

- *Do not overlap the lasagne sheets in the dish. Use a serrated knife to cut the lasagne sheets to fit the dish.*
- *To reheat lasagne (which cannot be stirred) in a microwave oven, cover and cook on LOW (40%) for 8–10 minutes to prevent the lasagne from toughening.*

VARIATION *Add vegetables of your choice to the pasta sauce. Cut them into similar sized pieces for speedy cooking.*

Big-flavour Bubble 'n' Squeak

SERVES 2

500 g mixed cooked vegetables (potatoes, pumpkin, broccoli, cauliflower, carrots)
salt and pepper, to taste
oil spray

CONVENTIONAL (10 MINUTES)

fork
bowl
non-stick frypan
wooden spoon
egg lifter
serving plate
knife

1. MASH the vegetables in the bowl with the fork until they are all roughly mixed together, and then season.
2. HEAT a lightly-oiled frypan over medium heat, add the vegetables and cook for 7 minutes, stirring four times during the cooking.
3. FLATTEN the vegetables into a large pancake, and invert onto a serving plate.

Slice, and serve.

HANDY MAN HINT *To 'feed the man meat', add chopped cooked sausage or meat to the vegies.*

VARIATION *Clean out the fridge, and use any vegetables you have available.*

Cauliflower Cheese Knockout

Serves 2

1 small cauliflower (500 g), roughly chopped
1 tsp water (microwave method only)
1 tsp chilli sauce
½ cup grated low-fat tasty cheese
1 cup white sauce (see page 150)
sweet paprika (for dusting)

CONVENTIONAL (35–40 MINUTES)

Preheat the oven to 200°C.

1 BRING a saucepan of water to the boil, and add the cauliflower. Cover, and cook over high heat for 8 minutes.
2 DRAIN the cauliflower, and place in the casserole dish. Place the white sauce in the jug, and stir in the chilli sauce and cheese. Pour the sauce over the cauliflower.
3 SPRINKLE with paprika, and bake in the middle of the oven for 20–25 minutes, or until the sauce is bubbling and golden.

Serve with a green salad.

chopping board
knife
large saucepan, and lid
sieve or colander
jug
ovenproof glass casserole dish
teaspoon
cup measure

MICROWAVE (12 MINUTES)

1 PLACE the cauliflower in the large microwave-safe container, and sprinkle with water. COVER, and cook on HIGH (100%) for 6 minutes. Remove from the oven, and drain away any liquid.
2 PLACE the white sauce in the jug, and stir in the chilli sauce and cheese. Pour the sauce over the cauliflower. Sprinkle with paprika.
3 COVER, and cook on HIGH (100%) for 3–4 minutes, until heated through.

Serve with a green salad.

chopping board
knife
large microwave-safe container, and lid
teaspoon
sieve or colander
spoon
jug

HANDY MAN HINT *Cooking cauliflower in the microwave oven eliminates odour from the kitchen.*

VARIATION *Add sliced chicken sausage or lean ham for a heartier meal.*

Corn on the Cob

Serves 2

2–4 fresh sweetcorn cobs
water (conventional method)
1 tbsp butter
1 tsp lemon juice
black pepper, freshly ground, to taste

CONVENTIONAL (20–25 MINUTES)

tablespoon
lemon juicer
teaspoon
large saucepan
small saucepan
spoon
serving tongs

1 REMOVE the leaves and silk from the cobs.
2 PLACE the water in a large saucepan, and bring to the boil. Add the cobs, and simmer over medium heat for 15–20 minutes. Drain.
3 MELT the butter in a small saucepan over low heat, and stir in the lemon juice.

Serve the cobs drizzled with the melted lemon butter, and add some freshly ground black pepper.

MICROWAVE (10–15 MINUTES)

tablespoon
lemon juicer
teaspoon
serving tongs
small microwave-safe container
spoon

1 PULL back the leaves (but do not remove), and remove the silk; then replace the leaves.
2 PLACE the cobs around the edge of the turntable, and cook on HIGH (100%) — 2 cobs, 7–8 minutes; 4 cobs, 8–9 minutes — turning them over halfway through the cooking time. Allow to stand for 1–2 minutes.
3 PLACE the butter in the microwave-safe dish, and cook, uncovered, on HIGH (100%) for 30 seconds. Stir in the lemon juice.

Serve the cobs drizzled with the melted lemon butter, and add some freshly ground black pepper.

VARIATION *To cook cobs on a barbecue, see page 54.*

Mushroom Mastery

'Life's too short to stuff a mushroom'
— Shirley Conran, Superwoman

Mushrooms are low in kilojoules, and are an excellent source of vitamin B and iron. There are many wholesome varieties to choose from. Most mushrooms on the market today are cultivated, and therefore available all year round. As there is little preparation involved before using them, experiment with some of the following varieties. Just wipe off any excess dirt, and trim the stalks before you cook them.

- Button mushrooms are mild in flavour; they can be eaten raw or added to salads or stir-fries.
- Field mushrooms have an open cup and a stronger flavour, and are perfect for frying in a little oil and serving on toast.
- Flat mushrooms are fully matured and one of the largest mushrooms; they have a strong flavour and good for barbecues or grills (see page 53).
- Oyster mushrooms (oyster shaped) originating in Asia have a delicate flavour. They should be cooked quickly, and are great for adding at the last minute to soups or stir-fries.

Dried mushrooms (such as shiitake and porcini) are also available; see hint below on rehydrating.

HANDY MAN HINTS

- *Choose mushrooms that are dry and firm, unwrinkled and evenly coloured.*
- *Do not store mushrooms in plastic, as they will sweat and deteriorate quickly.*
- *Mushrooms are 90% water, and will shrink when cooked conventionally.*
- *Microwaved mushrooms maintain their shape, size and flavour. Place them on a microwave-safe dinner plate, loosely cover with non-recycled paper towel, and cook on HIGH (100%) for 2 minutes. This way the dish you cook on doubles as the plate to eat from — saving washing up! The flavour of the mushrooms is enhanced by adding freshly cracked black pepper, olive oil, lemon juice and wine.*
- *To rehydrate dried mushrooms quickly in a microwave oven, place 4–6 mushrooms in a 4-cup microwave-safe glass jug and add 1 cup warm water. Cover with plastic wrap, leaving a small vent, and cook on HIGH (100%) for 4 minutes. Allow to stand for 5 minutes before draining.*

NETWORK

'A man without a woman is like a fish without a bicycle'

— Gloria Steinem (with apologies).

If you are a bloke who thinks fish is not filling or too smelly to cook, think again. Seafood has long been regarded as one of the healthiest foods from nature. Cooked with interesting spices and a side dish, or in the microwave oven, fish is flavoursome, odourless, and the ultimate fast food.

FIT TIPS

- Australians do not eat enough fish. Rich in omega-3 fats, fish is a great food for a healthy heart, and is relatively low in kilojoules to keep the body-fat levels down. One of the reasons we do not eat enough fish is ignorance in shopping, preparing and cooking of fresh fish.
- Don't forget that canned fish such as tuna, salmon and sardines are also very high in omega-3 fats and a good source of protein, and are particularly convenient and versatile.

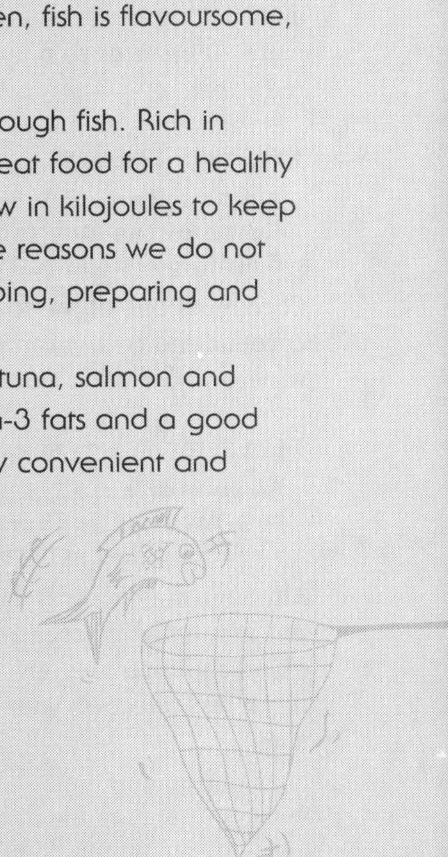

Grommet's Grub

Fish 'n' Chips (page 72)
Kiss Coleslaw (page 79)
Icecream Sundae Event (page 165)

Frozen crumbed fish fillets are a convenient way to enjoy fish. Look for varieties that are cooked in a minimum of polyunsaturated or monounsaturated oil.

Fit Fish Fast

Tuna Caesar (page 72)
Crusty bread roll
Dried Fruit and Nut Platter (page 196)

Caesar salad is traditionally a high-fat salad with egg, bacon, and a very creamy dressing. This version is just as tasty, but will leave you with room for plenty of fresh bread, and dried fruit to finish.

This is a good menu if you run at night after a hard day at work and cooking is not something you particularly enjoy. It will take a mere 10 minutes to prepare while you enjoy a well-earned glass of red wine!

Deep Blue

Big Red Herbed Tomato Soup (page 58)
Catch of the Day (page 73)
Goldfingers (page 197)

Coconut is one of the few plant foods high in saturated fats. Use coconut and coconut milk/cream sparingly, and choose the low-fat varieties now available.

Home Alone

Pizza Marinara (page 84)
Low-fat fruit yoghurt and canned fruit (e.g. peaches, pears or fruit salad in natural juice)

Although crayfish and lobster contain cholesterol, they are generally not consumed in large amounts or often enough to be of concern for blood-cholesterol levels. In addition, the cholesterol in food has much less effect on your blood cholesterol than the types of fat you eat.

How to Cook Fish

- *To fry fish:* Coat the fish lightly in flour, and cook with a small amount of polyunsaturated oil.
- *To grill fish:* Cover the grill tray with foil before cooking to keep the fish moist.
- *To pan-fry, grill or BBQ fish fillets:* Cook the fish with moderate heat for 2–3 minutes each side, depending on the thickness of the fillet, turning once only.
- *To bake whole fish (cleaned):* Score (cut) the flesh on either side to allow for even cooking. Cook for approximately 20 minutes per kilo.
- The fish is cooked when the flesh flakes easily at the thickest part.

How to Cook Fish in a Microwave Oven

This is an easy way to cook fish. Place the fillets or whole fish (cleaned) in a microwave-safe container. Cover loosely with plastic wrap or a lid. Cook on MEDIUM–HIGH (70%) power (for a 600–800W microwave oven), allowing 5 minutes per 500 g, or until the flesh flakes at its thickest part. Cooking times will be slightly shorter with higher wattage ovens.

FIT TIP

People with a high fish intake have a significantly lower incidence of heart disease, so eat fish or seafood at least twice a week for your heart's sake!

VARIATIONS FOR FLAVOUR

- *a squeeze of lime or lemon juice*
- *a sprinkling of fresh herbs and freshly ground black pepper*
- *a drizzle of dry white wine, and a sprinkling of toasted flaked almonds.*

Fish 'n' Chips

SERVES 2

4 crumbed frozen fish fillets
4 medium-sized washed potatoes (leave skin on), cut into wedges
2 tbsp olive oil
1 tsp paprika

CONVENTIONAL (30 MINUTES)

Preheat the oven to 225°C.

1 PLACE the fish fillets and potato wedges on the baking tray. Drizzle the potatoes with oil, and sprinkle with paprika.
2 BAKE in the middle of the oven for 20–25 minutes.

Serve with tartare sauce and lemon wedges, and a side salad of lettuce and cherry tomatoes.

chopping board
knife
metal baking tray
tablespoon
teaspoon

VARIATION *Sprinkle chips with dried herbs or garlic seasoning for extra flavour.*

Tuna Caesar

SERVES 2

1 pkt Caesar salad mix (or mesclun)
1 cup Caesar salad croutons (from the packet)
1 (425 g) can tuna, drained
2 large tomatoes, cut into 4 wedges
2 tbsp your favourite low-fat salad dressing (page 149)
1 tbsp shaved Parmesan cheese

CONVENTIONAL (7 MINUTES)

1 PLACE all the salad mix, croutons, tuna and tomato wedges in a large salad bowl, and toss with dressing.
2 SPRINKLE with the cheese.

Serve with a crisp bread roll.

bowl
cup measure
can opener
chopping board
knife
tablespoon

VARIATION *Substitute sliced sausages for the tuna.*

Catch of the Day

Serves 2

300 g flathead or trevally fillets, roughly chopped
½ red pepper, cut into thin 10 cm strips
4 spring onions, diagonally sliced
½ cup coconut milk (preferably low-fat)
1 tbsp curry powder

CONVENTIONAL (10–12 MINUTES)

chopping board
knife
can opener
cup measure
tablespoon
saucepan, and lid
wooden spoon

1 PLACE the fish, pepper and onions in the saucepan. Pour over the coconut milk, and stir through the curry powder.
2 COVER, and simmer (do not boil) over medium heat for 5–10 minutes, stirring halfway through the cooking time.

Serve with rice (pages 113, 114).

MICROWAVE (5 MINUTES)

chopping board
knife
can opener
cup measure
tablespoon
microwave-safe container, and lid

1 PLACE the fish, pepper and onions in the microwave-safe container. Pour over the coconut milk, and stir through the curry powder.
2 Cover, and cook on HIGH (100%) for 3 minutes, stirring halfway through the cooking time. Allow to stand for 1 minute.

Serve with rice (pages 113, 114).

HANDY MAN HINT

If you do not like the smell of fish cooking, use a microwave oven, and your kitchen will not smell like a fish shop.

VARIATIONS

Cook the rice in coconut milk and water for an Asian-style meal.

Pizza Marinara

SERVES 1

1 large pita bread
¼ cup Italian tomato pasta sauce
1 (290 g) can seafood marinara, drained, or 200 g fresh marinara mix
1 spring onion, chopped
¾ cup grated mozzarella cheese

CONVENTIONAL (10–12 MINUTES)

chopping board
knife
can opener
spoon
cup measure
metal baking tray

Preheat the oven to 220°C.

1 SPREAD the pita bread with tomato pasta sauce. Top with the marinara mix, onion, then the cheese.
2 PLACE the prepared pizza on the baking tray, and bake for 5–10 minutes until the base is crisp and the cheese has melted.

Serve with Greek Salad (page 84).

MICROWAVE (5 MINUTES)

chopping board
knife
can opener
spoon
cup measure
microwave-safe dinner plate
non-recycled paper towel

1 CRISP the pita bread by placing it on the turntable. Cook, uncovered, on HIGH (100%) for 2 minutes, turning it over halfway through the cooking time.
2 SPREAD the pita bread with tomato pasta sauce. Top with the marinara mix and onions, then the cheese.
3 PLACE two sheets of paper towel on an upturned dinner plate and place the pizza on top. Cook, uncovered, on HIGH (100%) for 1–1½ minutes until the cheese has melted.

Serve with Greek Salad (page 84).

HANDY MAN HINT

If a friend drops in, just double the recipe ingredients (and cooking time for the microwave method), and then go out and catch a movie together.

SALAD SUPERSTARS

'I never worry about diets; the only carrots that interest me are the number you get in diamonds'

— Mae West.

Salads have a bad reputation among many men, being viewed as rabbit food — which these days they are not! There are many substantial salad combinations, and salads are also an easy way to start a meal.

If you think there is too much shopping and chopping attached to salads, use ready-prepared salad mixes and toss them with a DIY or prepared dressing.

Salads are a good source of antioxidants that give protection from many health problems, such as cancer and heart disease — enough incentive to become a regular salad eater!

FIT TIPS Salads may seem a waste of space on the plate, but today's versions of salad are often meals in themselves, and offer easy and tasty ways of incorporating healthy vegetables. Use whatever lettuces and raw vegetables take your fancy, but opt for the low-oil varieties of dressings or just a little olive oil and lemon juice for a truly nutritious salad.

On the Greens

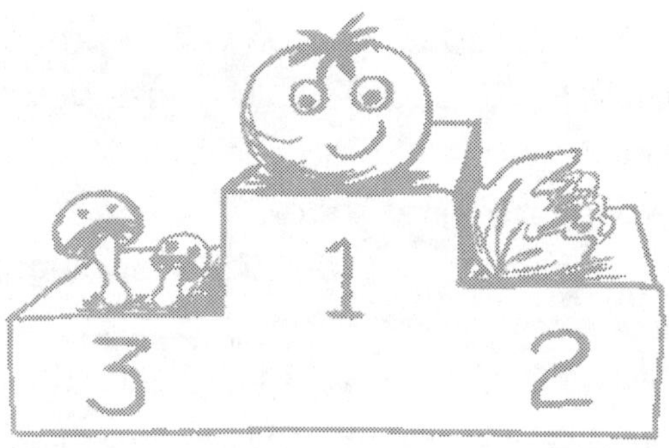

Silence-of-the-lamb Salad

Serves 1

300 g lean lamb strips
1 tbsp sweet chilli sauce
2 tsp Worcestershire sauce
100 g salad mix
½ green pepper, sliced into strips
½ salad onion, sliced into rings

CONVENTIONAL (10 MINUTES)

tablespoon
teaspoon
scales
chopping board
knife
non-stick frypan
wooden spoon
dinner plate

1 COMBINE the lamb, chilli sauce and Worcestershire sauce in the frypan, and cook over medium heat for 5 minutes, or until the lamb is cooked through, stirring at regular intervals. Allow to cool slightly.
2 PLACE the salad mix on a dinner plate, and top with the pepper and onion.
3 TOP the salad with the cooked lamb, and pour over any remaining juice for an easy dressing.

MICROWAVE (8 MINUTES)

tablespoon
teaspoon
scales
chopping board
knife
microwave-safe container
spoon
dinner plate

1 COMBINE the lamb, chilli sauce and Worcestershire sauce in the microwave-safe container. Cover, and cook on HIGH (100%) for 3 minutes, stirring halfway through the cooking time. Allow to stand for 2 minutes, and to cool slightly.
2 PLACE the salad mix on a dinner plate, and top with the pepper and onion.
3 TOP the salad with the cooked lamb, and pour over any remaining juice for an easy dressing.

HANDY MAN HINT

Sauces add flavour to meat, and also help to brown and tenderise it. If you leave the meat to marinate for a few hours before cooking, that will improve the texture and flavour of the meat.

VARIATION

Instead of the recipe vegetables, substitute any vegetables that you may have in your fridge.

Cucumber Raita Salad

1 long cucumber, peeled and finely sliced
1 tsp salt
1 tbsp chopped mint
200 g low-fat yoghurt

SERVES 2

chopping board
knife
bowl
spoon

CONVENTIONAL (20 MINUTES)

1 PLACE the cucumber slices in a bowl, and sprinkle the salt over it. Leave for 10–15 minutes.
2 POUR off any excess liquid, and drain the cucumber thoroughly, rinsing with cold water to remove most of the salt.
3 SPRINKLE the cucumber with the mint. Then stir in the yoghurt until the cucumber slices are evenly covered.

Serve with chicken satay or curries.

HANDY MAN HINT

The refreshing yoghurt mixture of raita creates a cooling contrast to a highly flavoured main dish.

Carbo-coleslaw

SERVES 2

250 g pkt coleslaw mix
1 (190 g) can kidney beans, drained
3 tbsp mayonnaise or dressing of your choice
2 spring onions, chopped
2 tsp chopped mint (optional)
black pepper, freshly ground, to taste

CONVENTIONAL (5 MINUTES)

1 COMBINE all the ingredients together in a large salad bowl, and mix through evenly.

Serve with meatloaf.

can opener
tablespoon
chopping board
knife
teaspoon

HANDY MAN HINT *Ready-to-go coleslaw and separate packs of dressing are available in packs at the supermarket.*

VARIATION *Add finely diced red and green peppers, and a chopped mango to the coleslaw, and season the mayonnaise with a pinch of mild curry powder to make a tropical coleslaw.*

KISS Coleslaw

SERVES 2

250 g pack coleslaw mix
3 tbsp low-fat mayonnaise
2 spring onions, chopped
2 tsp chopped mint (optional)
black pepper, freshly ground, to taste

CONVENTIONAL (5 MINUTES)

1 COMBINE all the ingredients together in a large salad bowl, and mix evenly.

Serve with fish or chops, or on top of potatoes.

tablespoon
chopping board
knife
teaspoon
large salad bowl
spoon

Top Tomato and Asparagus Salad

SERVES 2

2–3 cups cold water (conventional method); ¼ cup cold water (microwave)
1 bunch asparagus (12 spears), ends trimmed, and rinsed
3 slices lean ham, roughly chopped
2 (55 g) eggs, poached (page 18), drained and cooled
2 tomatoes, each cut into eight segments
1 tbsp oil and 1 tbsp lemon juice, mixed together with a fork (or shaken in a screwtop jar)

CONVENTIONAL (10 MINUTES)

chopping board
knife
tablespoon
cup or small screwtop jar
fork
non-stick frypan
2 dinner plates

1 PLACE the water in the frypan and bring to the boil. Add the asparagus, and cook over high heat for 1½ minutes. Cool under cold water, and drain.
2 FRY the ham in the pan over high heat for 4 minutes, until crisp. Drain on paper towel.
3 ASSEMBLE the salad by placing the tomato in a circle around the edge of two plates, and add the asparagus, ham and poached egg.

Drizzle with the dressing, and serve.

MICROWAVE (6 MINUTES)

chopping board
knife
tablespoon
cup or small screwtop jar
fork
shallow microwave-safe container, and lid
non-recycled paper towel
microwave-safe dinner plate
2 dinner plates

1 PLACE the asparagus in the microwave-safe container, and add ¼ cup water. Cover, and cook on HIGH (100%) for 1½ minutes. Cool under cold water, and drain.
2 Place one sheet of paper towel on a microwave-safe dinner plate, add the ham, and cover with another sheet of paper towel. Cook on HIGH (100%) for 3 minutes.
3 ASSEMBLE the salad by placing the tomato in a circle around the edge of two plates, and add the asparagus, ham and poached egg.

Drizzle with the dressing, and serve.

HANDY MAN HINTS

- *Buy unripe tomatoes and ripen them at home at room temperature, out of direct sunlight.*
- *Do not put tomatoes in the refrigerator since that affects both flavour and texture. This is a common mistake made by restaurants, greengroceries and takeaway outlets.*
- *Tomatoes are best eaten at room temperature, and the flavour can often be improved by slicing and sprinkling with a little castor sugar and salt a few minutes before serving.*
- *Tomatoes do not suffer significant nutritional loss in the canning process.*
- *Asparagus tips cook more quickly than the stalks. If you cook asparagus in a microwave oven, place the tips towards the centre, where they will cook more slowly.*

VARIATIONS *Until the last century known as love apples (from the French,* pommes d'amour*), tomatoes are versatile: they can be sliced, diced, stuffed, grilled, barbecued or added to salads or sandwiches.*

Honeyed Carrot Salad

SERVES 2–4

500 g carrots, sliced lengthwise
1 large orange, juiced
1 tbsp honey
1 tbsp chopped fresh parsley

CONVENTIONAL (8 MINUTES)

1 COMBINE all the ingredients in the saucepan.
2 COVER, and cook over low heat for 6–7 minutes, stirring once.

Serve as a warm salad, sprinkled with parsley.

chopping board
knife
lemon juicer
tablespoon
small saucepan, and lid

MICROWAVE (6 MINUTES)

1 COMBINE all the ingredients in the microwave-safe container.
2 COVER, and cook on HIGH (100%) for 4–5 minutes, stirring once.

Serve as a warm salad, sprinkled with parsley.

chopping board
knife
lemon juicer
tablespoon
small microwave-safe container and lid

Thai-style Pork Salad

Serves 2

1 tbsp oil
300 g lean new-fashioned pork schnitzel, pierced several times with a fork
2 tomatoes, sliced
1 large cucumber, sliced

Dressing
4 limes, juiced
1 tbsp soy sauce
1 tbsp seeded finely chopped chilli
1 tbsp mint

CONVENTIONAL (30 MINUTES)

tablespoon
chopping board
knife
lemon squeezer
small jug
non-stick frypan
egg lifter
2 dinner plates

1 HEAT the oil in the frypan for 30 seconds. Add the pork and cook over medium heat for 10 minutes, turning the meat over halfway through the cooking time.
2 CUT the pork into fine slices.
3 COMBINE all the dressing ingredients, pour over the meat. Leave to marinate for 15 minutes, if possible.

Place the tomato and cucumber slices on two dinner plates, and top with the dressed pork.

MICROWAVE (20–25 MINUTES)

tablespoon
chopping board
knife
lemon juicer
small jug
shallow microwave-safe container
non-recycled paper towel
2 dinner plates

1 PLACE the pork and oil in a microwave-safe container. Cover loosely with paper towel, and cook on HIGH (100%) for 3½ minutes, turning the meat over halfway through the cooking time.
2 ALLOW the meat to stand for 3 minutes. Cut the pork into fine slices. Combine all the dressing ingredients, and pour over the meat. Leave to marinate for 15 minutes, if possible.

Place the tomato and cucumber slices on two dinner plates, and top with the dressed pork.

HANDY MAN HINTS

- *Use lemons in the place of limes.*
- *Do not rub your eyes after chopping the chillies. Wash your hands thoroughly.*
- *Microwave hint: When turning meat over, also turn the outer edges towards the inside for even cooking.*

Peak-hour Potato and Sausage-sizzle Salad

Serves 2

4 low-fat chicken sausages, pierced three times with a fork
650 g Desiree (pink) potatoes, rinsed, and cut into 2 cm cubes
4 cups water
200 g frozen green baby beans
1 tbsp rosemary
2 tsp seeded mustard
2 tbsp light sour cream

CONVENTIONAL (20–25 MINUTES)

fork
chopping board
knife
tablespoon
teaspoon
non-stick frypan
egg lifter
saucepan, and lid
wooden spoon

1 PLACE the sausages in the frypan and cook over medium heat for 8–10 minutes, turning them over halfway through the cooking time. Remove the sausages, and cut them into 3 cm lengths.
2 PLACE the water in a saucepan and bring to the boil, add the potatoes, and cook over medium heat for 7–10 minutes until fork tender. Add the beans, and cook for 2 minutes. Drain the vegetables and return them to the saucepan. Stir in the rosemary, mustard, sour cream, and the cooked sausages.
3 COVER the saucepan, and cook over medium heat for 2 minutes.

Serve hot or cold.

MICROWAVE (12–15 MINUTES)

fork
chopping board
knife
tablespoon
teaspoon
large microwave-safe container, and lid
spoon

1 PLACE the sausages in the microwave-safe container. Cook, uncovered, on HIGH (100%) for 3 minutes. Remove the sausages, and cut them into 3 cm pieces.
2 PLACE the rinsed potatoes in the same container. Cover, and cook on HIGH (100%) for 5–6 minutes. Stir in the beans, rosemary, mustard, sour cream, and the cooked sausages.
3 COVER, and cook on HIGH (100%) for 2–3 minutes.

Serve hot or cold.

Greek Salad

SERVES 2

1 long cucumber, peeled and cut into 2 cm cubes
4 large tomatoes, cut into 2 cm cubes
100 g low-fat feta cheese, cut into 2 cm cubes
½ cup black pitted olives
1–2 tbsp fresh basil, chopped
2 tbsp oil, or the juice of an orange

chopping board
knife
potato peeler
cup measure
tablespoon
large serving bowl

CONVENTIONAL (5 MINUTES)

1 PLACE all the ingredients, except the oil or juice in the bowl.
2 MIX all the ingredients together evenly.
3 DRIZZLE with oil or orange juice.

Serve immediately.

HANDY MAN HINTS

- *To get more juice from an orange, place it in the microwave oven and cook on HIGH (100%) for 25 seconds before squeezing.*
- *Oranges freeze well.*
- *Vitamin C bonus: A regular orange could juice up your thinking. It is reported that high vitamin C intake may protect over-65s from memory loss. Get your vitamin C from any citrus fruits and from blackcurrants, strawberries, peppers, tomatoes, cauliflower and broccoli.*

Salad Tossed with Beans

SERVES 2

1 Iceberg lettuce, trimmed and cut into quarters
¾ cup water (conventional method); ¼ cup water (microwave)
200 g green beans, topped and tailed
½ cup French dressing (page 00)
4 spring onions, sliced diagonally

CONVENTIONAL (5 MINUTES)

chopping board
knife
cup measure
salad bowl
medium-sized saucepan
colander
spoon

1 PLACE the lettuce in the salad bowl.
2 PLACE the water in the saucepan and bring to the boil. Add the beans, and cook over medium heat for 2 minutes only. Cool the beans under cold running water, then drain them and transfer them to the salad bowl.
3 SCATTER with the onions, drizzle with the dressing, and toss.

Serve with slices of Macho Meat Loaf (page 101).

MICROWAVE (5 MINUTES)

chopping board
knife
cup measure
salad bowl
small microwave-safe container, and lid
colander
spoon

1 PLACE the lettuce in the salad bowl.
2 POUR ¼ cup water into the microwave-safe container. Add the beans. Cover, and cook on HIGH (100%) for 2 minutes. Cool the beans under cold running water, then drain them and transfer them to the serving bowl.
3 SCATTER with the onions, drizzle with the dressing, and toss.

Serve with slices of Macho Meat Loaf (page 101).

HANDY MAN HINT

To top and tail fresh beans: use a sharp knife to trim 2 mm off each end of the beans.

Rabbits' Food

Salad greens may be too green for you, but these days there are twelve kinds of fresh lettuces to choose from at the supermarkets. Why not buy and try some of the following varieties?

Green with Envy Salads

Iceberg: tightly-furled, light-green all-rounder for most meals.

Endive: curly-leaved, slightly bitter lettuce, good with Italian food.

Radicchio: red, curly-leafed lettuce, quite peppery in flavour; serve with barbecued meats grilled with olive oil.

Mixture of lettuces (mesclun): includes oak leaf lettuce, spinach leaves, radicchio, endive, and many other salad leaves.

Baby English spinach leaves: buy them washed, and ready to go, add a French or DIY dressing, or throw into a noodle dish, stir-fries or soups; great with any Kiss the Chef meals (pages 141–6).

A green salad can be much more than plain lettuce. If you do not like washing and chopping, try the ready-to-go salad in the packs. They have no additives, and are natural, crisp and crunchy.

Try eating them straight, or toss them with your favourite dressing. Salads are virtually fat free, and low in kilojoules. There is no effort involved in opening a bag to make eating easy.

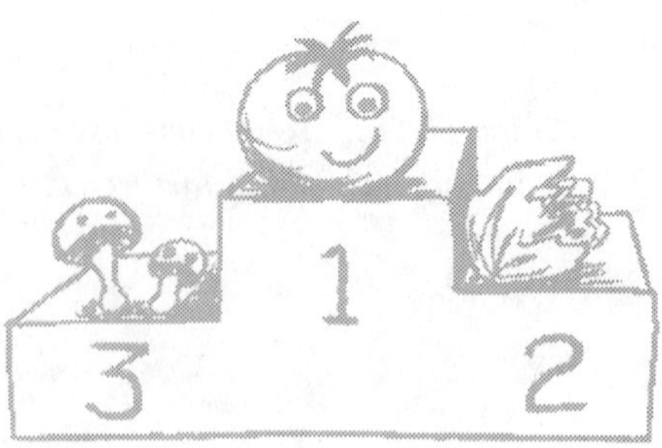

WHERE'S THE MEAT?

'I guess my taste in food has grown a lot over the past couple of years. When I was 17 or 18, it was basically meat and a few vegies. Now I like to try most things, and really enjoy Thai, Indian and Mexican cuisines'

— Steve Waugh.

If you are basically a meat bloke, keep the balance on the plate rather than just devouring copious quantities of meat. Vegies, rice or pasta should take up three-quarters of the plate, and meat the other quarter.

FIT TIPS

- 'Feed the man meat' was an advertising cry of the 1970s; the 1990s' message is probably more along the lines of 'Feed the man less meat'! Not *no* meat, but smaller portions, leaner meat, and less fat in the preparation.
- Red meat is an excellent source of iron, zinc and protein — all important for work, rest and play, but large quantities can be a problem for both cholesterol and waist measurements! Lean red meat has very little 'marbling or streaking' of fat through it, and all visible fat is trimmed where possible. The National Heart Foundation 'tick of approval' is a useful guide.

Blokes Around the Barbie

Stab-pass Beef Skewers (page 92)
Sausages for SNAGS (page 93)
Lemony Lamb Racks (page 94)
Burgers for Blokes (pages 95–7)
- **Oz Burger** (page 95)
- **Mediterranean-style Burger** (page 96)
- **Indian Burger** (page 97)
- **Asian Kofta Burgers** (page 127)

BBQ Corn on the Cob (page 54)
BBQ Vegetables (page 53)
Greek Salad (page 84)
Crusty bread
Seasonal Fruit 'n' Nut Platter (page 194)

Barbecues are a great Aussie eating tradition. A healthy barbecue should have a good balance of lean meat, fresh vegetables or salad, and bread, with seasonal fruit to finish. Avoid the trap of a barbecue based on meat — make sure there are plenty of carbohydrates to fill up on. Barbecuing is a great way of cooking meat, as it lets any fat drip out during the cooking — just keep the added oil to a minimum.

Pumping Iron

Steak My Way (page 98)
Mountains of Mash (page 60)
Green peas
Canned peaches, with low-fat Fromage Frais

Select small steaks, and fill up on the 'mountains of mash', peas and fruit. This is a great recovery meal after a big day of exercise.

Scozzers' Snags

Super Sausage Sizzle (page 99)
Fried Rice (page 100)
Low-fat icecream, with canned fruit salad

Sausages are normally a high-fat, high-salt product. In response to consumer demand many major supermarkets and butchers have now introduced low-fat, low-salt sausages, which are surprisingly delicious.

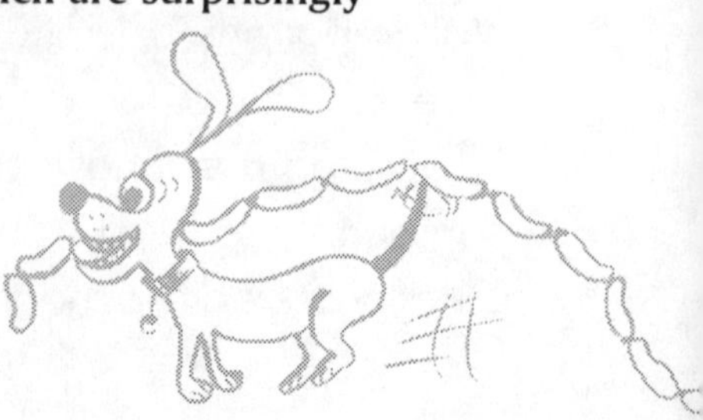

Use Your Loaf

Macho Meat Loaf (page 101)
Corn on the cob (page 54)
Salad Tossed with Beans (page 85)
Carbo-coleslaw (page 79) **and DIY Dressing** (page 149)
Fast-track Banana Custard (page 163)

Meat loaf is such a simple favourite to make. Add some sweetcorn, rice, pasta or potatoes for a high-carbo meal.

The Frying Game

Veal Schnitzel Veronica (page 102)
Baked potato (page 56)
'Bowled' Berry Pudding (page 160)

Whenever a food is fried in oil its fat content increases. This is a relatively healthy version of veal schnitzel, using lean veal and a little olive oil.

Lounge Lizards

Lamb Chops with Avocado Salsa (page 103)
Mountains of Mash (page 60)
Green beans
Perfect Pancakes (page 162)

Avocado is a highly nutritious fruit with loads of vitamins and minerals, but it is also high in mono-unsaturated fats. This means that it is high in kilojoules (if you are watching your weight), but is OK for cholesterol-watchers.

Just Stirring

Beef Stir-fry All-rounder (page 104)
Hokkein Noodles (page 43)
Grapes

Add chestnuts to your stir-fries to boost your vitamin E intake without overdoing the fat. Always choose unroasted, unsalted nuts.

In summer freeze whole seedless grapes for an iced dessert, or for a healthy 'snack attack'.

Ribs to Spare

Pork Spare Ribs (page 105)
Fried Rice (page 100)

Pork was once considered a high-fat meat, but the 'New-fashioned Pork' available today is lean, and a great source of protein, B vitamins, iron and zinc.

Cruisy Casserole

One-pot Beef Casserole (page 106)
Chocolate Cake (page 159)

There's nothing better on a cold night after training or work than a steaming casserole and piles of rice or potato. This dish is a rich source of iron and zinc, both important minerals for peak performance and good health.

Try herbed or spicy sausages:

Boerworst: coarse, thick beef sausage with coriander seeds.

Bratwurst: fine-textured thick or thin pork or beef sausage, with a spicy and mild flavour.

Chevapcici: coarse-minced skinless pork, lamb or beef sausage.

Chipolatas: very thin, small pork sausages, often made with other flavours.

Chorizo: thick, spicy pork sausage.

Ctechino: very thick, coarse pork sausage with a subtly spiced skin.

Cumberland: thick curly pork sausage with sage and marjoram.

Debreciner (debriezener): spicy smoked pork sausage.

English pork: thick or thin, finely minced pork sausage with a little seasoning.

Frankfurter: thin, fine-textured smoked beef, veal and pork sausages; saveloys are skinless frankfurters.

Kransky: medium to coarse, thick pork and beef sausages, often with cheese.

Toulouse: coarse, thick pork sausage, cooked and smoked.

Weisswurst: fine minced, pre-cooked, thick veal and pork sausages.

FIT TIP *Sausages are a very high-fat food. Look for low-fat options, or use them for indulgences only.*

How to Roast Beef — the Main Event

Serves 4

800 g silverside, trimmed of excess fat and cut into an even shape
¼ cup wholegrain mustard
black pepper, freshly ground, to taste

CONVENTIONAL (1 HOUR)

Preheat the oven to 250°C.

1 SPREAD the mustard evenly over the meat with the knife. Place the meat in the baking tray in the middle of the oven, and bake for 45 minutes.
2 ALLOW to stand for 5–10 minutes in a warm place, before carving into eight slices.

Serve with vegetables (pages 49–52).

chopping board
knife
cup measure
table knife
metal baking tray
carving dish
carving knife and fork

MICROWAVE (25–30 MINUTES)

1 SPREAD the mustard evenly over the meat with the knife. Place the meat on top of an upturned dinner plate within a shallow microwave-safe container.
2 COVER loosely with paper towel, and cook on MEDIUM–HIGH (70–80%) for 15 minutes.
3 COVER with foil, and allow to stand for 5–10 minutes before carving into eight slices.

Serve with vegetables (pages 49–52).

chopping board
knife
cup measure
table knife
microwave-safe dinner plate
non-recycled paper towel
foil
carving dish
carving knife and fork

HANDY MAN HINTS

- *Evenly-shaped cuts of meat cook best.*
- *Roasted meats, in particular, carve best when 'rested'. Remove the meat from the source of heat, and place on a board; cover, and keep the meat warm for 10–12 minutes. The juices will stop running, and return to the centre (now the source of greatest heat). Carving will be easier, and the meat tenderer. This also applies to steak.*
- *Check that your knife is sharp enough for carving (see page 8).*
- *Use leftover sliced beef in a sandwich (see page 34).*

Stab-pass Beef Skewers

SERVES 4

280 g lean rump/porterhouse (fat removed), chopped into cubes
8 cherry tomatoes
4 yellow squash, halved (or mushrooms)
¼ cup pickled onions
¼ cup stuffed olives (optional)

CONVENTIONAL (20 MINUTES)

chopping board
knife
cup measure
long metal skewers
tongs or oven gloves

1 THREAD the meat, tomatoes, squash, onions and olives onto skewers. Repeat twice for each skewer.
2 PLACE the skewers on a preheated barbecue grill, and cook over high heat for 10 minutes, turning the skewers regularly.

*Remove the skewers, and serve with **Peak-hour Potato Sausage-sizzle Salad** (page 83).*

HANDY MAN HINTS

- *To tenderise the meat, marinate it in ½ cup red wine, seasoned with 2 cloves fresh garlic, and a spring onion and/or 1 tsp rosemary. You can do this ahead of time, and take it to a barbecue in a sealed container.*
- *Garlic cloves are easy to peel if you place the cloves in a microwave oven, and heat on HIGH (100%) for 10 seconds each. The garlic will then slip out of the skin.*

VARIATION *Use your favourite sauce as a marinade.*

Sausages for SNAGS

SERVES 2

1 tbsp tomato sauce and 1 tbsp Worcestershire sauce, combined
6 low-fat sausages, pierced 3 times with a fork

CONVENTIONAL (12 MINUTES)

tablespoon
small bowl (or screwtop jar)
pastry brush
tongs

1 PLACE the sausages on a preheated barbecue grill, and brush with half of the combined sauces. Cook for 5 minutes.
2 TURN the sausages over, and brush them with remaining sauces. Cook for a further 5 minutes.

Slice the sausages, and serve in a Caesar salad (page 73).

MICROWAVE (5 MINUTES)

tablespoon
small bowl (or screwtop jar)

1 PIERCED sausages will cook quickly in the microwave if placed on the edge of the turntable. Brush the sausages with the combined sauce before cooking. Two thin sausages will take 2–3 minutes on HIGH (100%); four will take 4 minutes on HIGH (100%).
2 Leave to stand for 1 minute before serving.

Slice the sausages, and serve in a Caesar salad (page 73).

HANDY MAN HINTS

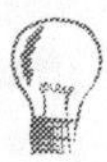

How to cook perfect snags:

- *Remove the sausages from the fridge 30 minutes before cooking.*
- *Cook in a non-stick frypan over low heat to prevent natural skins splitting. Keep rolling them over to ensure even browning.*
- *If you are barbecuing them, blanch them first in boiling water to seal the skins and prevent them bursting on contact with heat. Blanched sausages can be cooked over higher heat. This method is especially recommended for thick sausages.*

FIT TIP

Many supermarkets now have low-fat varieties of sausages. Look for those with less than 10% fat.

Lemony Lamb Racks

Serves 2

2 racks lamb (3 cutlets each), trimmed of all fat and sinew, and slit between each cutlet (but not right through).
¼ cup oil
2 medium-sized lemons, juiced
2 tsp rosemary
salt and paper, to taste

chopping board
knife
cup measure
lemon juicer
teaspoon
large bowl
whisk or fork
tongs
absorbent paper

CONVENTIONAL (45 MINUTES)

1 WHISK the oil, lemon juice, herbs and seasoning together in a large bowl, and add the racks. Leave to marinate for 30 minutes.
2 PLACE the racks on the hottest part of the preheated barbecue grill and cook, fat-side down, for 8–10 minutes.
3 TURN the racks over, and cook over high heat for a further 5 minutes.

Serve with spicy barbecue vegetables (page 53).

HANDY MAN HINTS

- *Lamb racks cook evenly and quickly when the meat is cut down well between the bones.*
- *To cook individual cutlets: place separate marinated lamb cutlets on the hottest part of the barbecue, and cook for 3 minutes on each side. Drain on absorbent paper.*

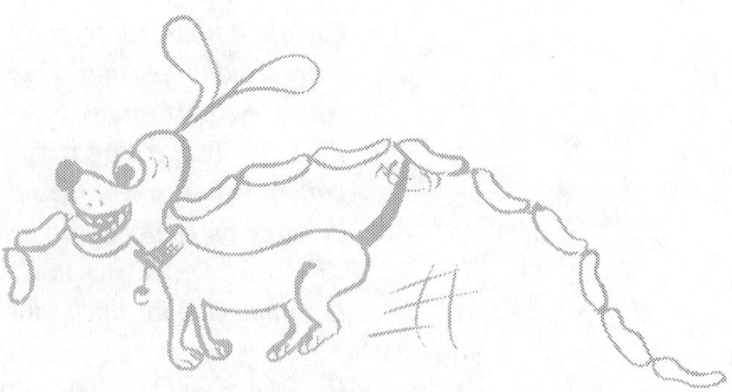

Burgers for Blokes

Burgers are a great way to get variety with meat! Just make sure that you select the leanest mince meat from your butcher or supermarket, and eat plenty of bread and salad with your burgers.

Oz Burger

Serves 2–4

250 g lean minced beef
1 cup grated low-fat cheese
2 tbsp tomato sauce
2 slices canned pineapple, chopped
4 wholemeal burger buns, cut in half (toasted, if preferred)
Iceburg lettuce leaves

CONVENTIONAL (15 MINUTES)

mixing bowl
fork (or plastic bag; see hint, page 96)
cup measure
tablespoon
can opener
chopping board
knife
non-stick frypan
egg lifter

1 COMBINE the mince, cheese, sauce and pineapple in the bowl, mixing thoroughly. Shape into four burgers.
2 HEAT the frypan over medium heat, and add the burgers. Cook over medium heat for 6 minutes, turning them over halfway through the cooking time.

Place the lettuce leaves and burger inside each bun to serve.

VARIATIONS

- *If you would like an egg in your burger, heat an egg ring on the barbecue and crack in an egg, turning it after 2–3 minutes. If you do not have an egg ring, make a hole in the centre of a slice of bread and use this as an egg ring (in toast!).*
- *Satay-flavoured burgers can be made by adding ¼ cup satay sauce to the minced beef. Serve with rice in place of a bun.*

Mediterranean-style Burger

SERVES 2–4

250 g lean minced beef
3 tbsp tomato pasta sauce
20 g pitted black olives, chopped roughly
10 g capers (optional)
lettuce greens (try endive)
4 burger buns, cut in half (toasted, if preferred)

CONVENTIONAL (15 MINUTES)

mixing bowl
fork (or plastic bag; see hint, below)
tablespoon
scales
chopping board
knife
non-stick frypan
egg lifter

1 COMBINE all the ingredients, except the lettuce and buns, in the bowl. When the mixture is evenly combined, shape into four burgers.
2 HEAT the frypan over medium heat. Add the burgers, and cook over medium heat for 6 minutes, turning them over halfway through the cooking time.

Place some lettuce and a burger in each bun to serve.

MICROWAVE (8 MINUTES)

mixing bowl
fork (or plastic bag; see hint, below)
tablespoon
scales
chopping board
knife
microwave-safe dinner plate
non-recycled paper towel

1 COMBINE all the ingredients, except the lettuce and buns, in the bowl. When the mixture is evenly combined, shape into four burgers.
2 PLACE two sheets of paper towel on a dinner plate, and put the burgers on top. Cover with two sheets of paper towel, and cook on HIGH (100%) for 4 minutes.

Place some lettuce and a burger in each bun to serve.

HANDY MAN HINTS

- *To mix mince: simply place a plastic bag over your hand first — you will find it easier and cleaner to mix this way.*
- *Hamburger junkies can take advantage of bulk specials by freezing fresh lean beef mince in 500 g portions in flat packages (to defrost or thaw quickly).*

Indian Burger

SERVES 2–4

250 g lean beef mince
1 tsp mild curry powder
½ tsp cinnamon
1 tsp dried coriander
½ small cucumber, chopped
4 wholemeal burger buns, cut in half (toasted, if preferred)
mixed lettuce pieces

CONVENTIONAL (15 MINUTES)

1 COMBINE all the ingredients, except the lettuce and buns, in the bowl. When the mixture is evenly combined, shape into four burgers.
2 HEAT the frypan over medium heat. Add the burgers, and cook over medium heat for 6 minutes, turning them over halfway through the cooking time.

Place some lettuce and a burger in each bun to serve.

mixing bowl
fork (or plastic bag; see hint, page 96)
teaspoon
chopping board
knife
non-stick frypan
egg lifter

MICROWAVE (8 MINUTES)

1 COMBINE all the ingredients, except the lettuce and buns, in the bowl. When the mixture is evenly combined, shape into four burgers.
2 PLACE two sheets of paper towel on a dinner plate, and put burgers on top. Cover with two sheets of paper towel, and cook on HIGH (100%) for 4 minutes.

Place some lettuce and a burger in each bun to serve.

mixing bowl
fork (or plastic bag; see hint, page 96)
teaspoon
chopping board
knife
microwave-safe dinner plate
non-recycled paper towel

HANDY MAN HINT

Allow plenty of time for the mince to cook through — cook the burgers for about 3–4 minutes each side, depending on the thickness of the burgers. Test by cutting one open to check the colour, and cook a little longer if the meat inside still looks pink.

Steak My Way

SERVES 2

1 tbsp oil or cooking oil spray
2 lean rump steaks (400 g), at room temperature
2 (55 g) eggs
1 tbsp pesto or 1 tbsp tomato or taco or Worcestershire sauce

tablespoon
non-stick frypan
egg lifter
warmed plate

CONVENTIONAL (12½ MINUTES)

1 HEAT the oil in the frypan over low heat for 30 seconds.
2 PLACE the steak in the pan, turn up the heat, and cook for 8 minutes, turning the steak over halfway through the cooking time. Remove the steak, and place it on a warmed plate.
3 CRACK the eggs into the pan, and cook over low heat for 2 minutes. Turn them over, and cook for a further 2 minutes.

Serve on top of the steak with one of the sauces.

HANDY MAN HINTS

- *You can use silverside, eye steak or oyster blade steak in place of rump steak. Check the meat is lean enough to give a good supply of nutrients, such as iron and zinc, without the unnecessary fat.*
- *Use cooking oil spray in place of oil.*

Super Sausage Sizzle

SERVES 2

4 (250 g) low-fat sausages, pierced 3 times with a fork
cold water to cover
150 g button mushrooms, quartered
100 g green beans, halved (fresh or frozen)
½ cup combined tomato and Worcestershire sauces
½ cup water
1 tbsp cornflour blended with 1 tbsp water

CONVENTIONAL (30 MINUTES)

fork
chopping board
knife
cup measure
tablespoon
small bowl
medium-sized saucepan
colander
wooden spoon

1 PUT the sausages and water in the saucepan, and bring them slowly to the boil. Drain the sausages, and slice into 1 cm rounds.
2 COMBINE the sausages, mushrooms, beans, sauces and water in the saucepan, cover and simmer over medium heat for 20 minutes, stirring several times.
3 ADD the cornflour, and continue to simmer, uncovered, until the sauce has thickened, stirring two or three times during cooking.

Serve over cooked rice (pages 113, 114).

MICROWAVE (12 MINUTES)

fork
chopping board
knife
cup measure
tablespoon
small bowl
non-recycled paper towel
large microwave-safe container, and lid
spoon

1 PLACE the sausages on the turntable, and cover with paper towel. Cook on HIGH (100%) for 1½ minutes.
2 SLICE the sausages into 1 cm rounds, and place them in a large microwave-safe container with the mushrooms, beans, sauces and water. Cover, and cook on HIGH (100%) for 4 minutes.
3 ADD the cornflour. Cover, and cook on HIGH (100%) for 1 minute. Allow to stand for 2 minutes, then stir.

Serve over cooked rice (pages 113, 114).

VARIATION *Add a can of mixed beans for an energy boost, or chopped grilled lean bacon for extra flavour.*

Fried Rice

SERVES 2

1 tbsp oil
150 g carrots, finely chopped
150 g broccoli florets
2 tbsp soy sauce
2½ cups cooked rice, at room temperature (pages 113, 114)

CONVENTIONAL (10 MINUTES)

tablespoon
scales
chopping board
knife
cup measure
non-stick frypan
egg lifter
wooden spoon

1 HEAT the oil in the frypan over medium heat for 1 minute.
2 ADD the carrots, broccoli and soy sauce, and mix through evenly. Cook over medium heat for 5 minutes, stirring constantly.
3 ADD the rice, and mix through evenly. Cook for a further 3 minutes to reheat the rice.

Serve as a side dish.

MICROWAVE (10 MINUTES)

tablespoon
scales
chopping board
knife
cup measure
large microwave-safe container, and lid

1 COMBINE the oil, carrots, broccoli and soy sauce in the microwave-safe container, and mix evenly.
2 COVER, and cook on HIGH (100%) for 5 minutes, stirring halfway through the cooking time.
3 ADD the rice, and mix through evenly. Cover, and cook on HIGH (100%) for 2 minutes to reheat the rice.

Serve as a side dish.

VARIATIONS *Add bean shoots, or snow peas, or canned baby corn for Chinese-style fried rice.*

Macho Meat Loaf

SERVES 2

2 tbsp chutney
1 tbsp Worcestershire sauce
1 small red pepper (or celery or carrot), cut into 1 cm cubes
½ cup breadcrumbs
400 g lean beef mince

CONVENTIONAL (40–50 MINUTES)

Preheat the oven to 180°C.

1 COMBINE the chutney, Worcestershire sauce and pepper in the frypan over medium heat for 2–3 minutes, or until the pepper has softened.
2 REMOVE from the heat, and stir in the breadcrumbs and mince, and mix until well combined. Shape the meat mixture into a log, 15 cm × 12 cm. Place on the baking tray. Bake, uncovered, for 30–45 minutes.
3 ALLOW to stand for 10 minutes.

Serve with a salad or vegies.

tablespoon
chopping board
knife
cup measure
non-stick frypan
wooden spoon
metal baking tray
carving plate
carving knife and fork

MICROWAVE (12–15 MINUTES)

1 COMBINE the chutney, Worcestershire sauce and pepper in the microwave-safe container. Cook, uncovered, on HIGH (100%) for 1 minute.
2 STIR in the breadcrumbs and mince, and mix until well combined. Shape the meat mixture into a log, 15 cm × 12 cm. Place the log on two sheets of paper towel on the dinner plate, and cover with two more sheets of paper towel. Cook on HIGH (100%) for 10 minutes.
3 ALLOW to stand for 10 minutes, then slice.

Serve with a salad or vegies.

tablespoon
chopping board
knife
cup measure
large microwave-safe container
spoon
microwave-safe dinner plate
non-recycled paper towel

HANDY MAN HINTS

- *Meat loaf can be frozen, used in sandwiches, reheated in the microwave, or taken to a picnic.*
- *Allowing the meatloaf, whether cooked conventionally or in the microwave, to rest for 10 minutes before serving makes it firmer and easier to slice.*

Veal Schnitzel Veronica

Serves 2

2 veal or pork schnitzels (400 g)
2 eggs, lightly beaten
1 cup dried breadcrumbs
2 tsp mixed dried herbs
1½ tbsp olive oil

CONVENTIONAL (12 MINUTES)

mixing bowl
egg beater or fork
cup measure
teaspoon
meat mallet (or a large unopened can, and plastic wrap to cover the meat)
non-stick frypan
egg lifter
absorbent paper

1 BEAT the schnitzels with the meat mallet until they are an *even thickness*. Mix the herbs and breadcrumbs in a shallow dish. Pour the beaten egg into another shallow container.
2 DIP the schnitzels into the egg until they are completely covered, and then into the herbed breadcrumbs, coating them completely.
3 HEAT the oil in the frypan over medium heat, and cook the schnitzels for 4 minutes; turn them and cook for another 2 minutes on the other side or until golden brown. Drain on absorbent paper.

Serve with Cucumber Raita Salad (page 78) and a wedge of lemon.

HANDY MAN HINT *Place the schnitzels between sheets of plastic wrap before beating them with the mallet or can to prevent the meat from being torn to shreds while making them an even thickness.*

VARIATION *Add 1 tbsp Parmesan cheese to the breadcrumbs for a flavour change.*

Lamb Chops with Avocado Salsa

SERVES 2

6–8 lamb chops, trimmed of all fat

Salsa

1 ripe avocado
juice of 1 small lemon
½ red onion, finely chopped
1 dash tabasco sauce
salt and pepper, to taste

CONVENTIONAL (15 MINUTES)

chopping board
knife
lemon juicer
non-stick frypan
egg lifter
mixing bowl
fork

1 COOK the lamb chops in the frypan over medium heat for 4–5 minutes each side.
2 COMBINE all the salsa ingredients in the bowl, and mash them together with a fork until evenly mixed.
3 TOP the cooked lamb chops with the salsa.

Serve with white or red beans (pages 109–10).

HANDY MAN HINT

If you do not have a non-stick frypan, use a sheet of recycled paper towel as a brush to lightly oil your pan.

VARIATION

Top with Worcestershire sauce or Tomato Sauce Supreme (see page 151).

Beef Stir-fry All-rounder

SERVES 2

2 tsp oil
300 g lean beef strips
250 g stir-fry vegetables (e.g. carrots, onions, broccoli florets), fresh or frozen
¼ cup stir-fry sauce
1 tbsp peanuts or cashews, unroasted and unsalted

CONVENTIONAL (12 MINUTES)

teaspoon
scales
cup measure
tablespoon
non-stick frypan
wooden spoon
spoon

1 MELT the oil in the frypan over low heat. Add the beef and stir-fry over low heat for 5 minutes.
2 REMOVE the beef to a warm plate, and cover it with paper towel. Add the vegetables to the pan, and stir-fry for 3–5 minutes.
3 ADD the cooked meat and the sauce to the pan, and heat through.

Stir in the nuts before serving on rice or noodles (pages 112–14).

MICROWAVE (10 MINUTES)

teaspoon
scales
cup measure
tablespoon
large microwave-safe container
spoon
warmed plate
non-recyclable paper towel

1 PLACE the oil in the microwave-safe container. Cook, uncovered, on HIGH (100%) for 30 seconds. Stir in the beef, and cook, uncovered, on HIGH (100%) for 3 minutes, stirring halfway through the cooking time. Drain the beef, and place on a warmed plate and cover it with paper towel.
2 ADD the vegetables to the container. Cook, uncovered, on HIGH (100%) for 3 minutes, stirring halfway through the cooking time.
3 ADD the cooked meat and the sauce, and cook on HIGH (100%) for 1½ minutes.

Stir in the nuts before serving on rice or noodles (pages 112–14).

HANDY MAN HINTS

- *Cook the rice in the microwave oven while you are cooking the stir-fry on the stovetop.*
- *Place leftovers in a sealed container, and take to work for microwave reheating.*

Pork Spare Ribs

SERVES 2

4 pork spare rib cutlets (700 g), trimmed of excess fat
½ cup plum or soy or sweet 'n' sour sauce

CONVENTIONAL (55 MINUTES)

chopping board
knife
cup measure
deep dish
metal baking tray

Preheat the oven to 220°C.

1 PLACE the prepared ribs in a deep dish, and pour over the sauce. Leave to marinate for 30 minutes.
2 PLACE the spare ribs on the baking tray, and bake for 15–20 minutes.
3 DRIZZLE with any remaining sauce. Allow to stand for 2 minutes.

Serve with rice (pages 113, 114).

MICROWAVE (45 MINUTES)

chopping board
knife
cup measure
deep dish
microwave-safe rack
spoon
non-recycled paper towel

1 PLACE the prepared ribs in a deep dish, and pour over the sauce. Leave to marinate for 30 minutes.
2 PLACE the spare ribs on a microwave-safe rack, with the meat towards the outer edge and the bones towards the centre.
3 DRIZZLE the ribs with any remaining sauce. Cover loosely with paper towel, and cook on HIGH (100%) for 10 minutes, turning the ribs over halfway through the cooking time. Allow to stand for 2 minutes.

Serve with rice (pages 113, 114).

HANDY MAN HINT

Leave spare ribs marinating for 2 hours, to tenderise the meat.

One-pot Beef Casserole

SERVES 2

400 g lean beef steak (rump, sirloin or fillet)
250 g mixed frozen vegetables
1–2 stock cubes, crumbled
250 ml V8 vegetable juice, hot
2 tbsp chopped parsley

CONVENTIONAL (1 HOUR)

scales
chopping board
knife
tablespoon
meat mallet (or a large unopened can, and plastic wrap to cover the steak)
fork
can opener
casserole dish, and lid
spoon

Preheat the oven to 200°C.

1 BEAT the steak with a meat mallet until it is an even thickness. Pierce the steak five times with a fork, and cut the steak into 2½ cm cubes. Place the meat cubes in a casserole dish with the vegetables, stock cube and V8 juice. Mix evenly.
2 COVER, and bake for 45 minutes until the meat is soft when pierced with a fork. Stir once.
3 ALLOW to stand for 5 minutes.

Sprinkle with parsley, and serve with mashed potatoes (page 60).

MICROWAVE (25 MINUTES)

scales
chopping board
knife
tablespoon
meat mallet (or a large unopened can, and plastic wrap to cover the steak)
fork
can opener
microwave-safe container, and lid
spoon

1 BEAT the steak with a meat mallet until it is an even thickness. Pierce the steak five times with a fork, and cut the steak into 2½ cm cubes. Place the cubed meat in a microwave-safe container.
2 COOK, uncovered, on HIGH (100%) for 3 minutes, stirring halfway through the cooking time. Drain off any excess liquid.
3 ADD the frozen vegetables, stock cube and V8 juice. Cover, and cook on HIGH (100%) for 10 minutes, stirring halfway through the cooking time. Allow to stand for 5 minutes.

Sprinkle with parsley, and serve with mashed potatoes (page 145).

HANDY MAN HINT

Athletes may be at high risk of low iron levels because of an inadequate diet or an increased rate of iron loss. Try this casserole with an entree of oysters for an energy booster (page 145).

Beating the Bypass

'One should eat to live, not live to eat'

— Molière (1622–73).

For any average less-than-athletic, '14-hour-a-day' man, running once or twice a week (sometimes), the benefits of eating less meat and fats, and more vegetables, pasta and rice are hard to ignore.

Cardio-watch fit tips

- Despite the good news that fewer people now have high cholesterol, and deaths from coronary heart disease are falling, heart disease is still a major killer of men in Australia. You do have some control over this, however, as many of the risk factors for heart disease are preventable. The food you eat, for example, can help keep your blood cholesterol, blood pressure and weight under control.
- One of the key dietary factors is to watch your fat intake. Not only should we all be reducing dietary fat, but it is also important to replace saturated fat with mono- and polyunsaturated fats.

Saturated fats

Many of the saturated fats are known to increase blood cholesterol and blood clots, and therefore increase the risk of heart disease.

These types of fats are found in full-cream milk, cheese, butter, cream, fatty meats and poultry, sausages and many processed foods.

Mono-unsaturated fats

When you replace saturated fats with these fats in your diet, they can have a very positive effect on your blood cholesterol (by lowering the 'bad' LDL-cholesterol and increasing the 'good' HDL-cholesterol). However, they are just as high in kilojoules, and therefore just as fattening as any other type of fat.

Foods high in mono-unsaturated fats include olive oil, canola oil, olives, peanuts and avocados.

Polyunsaturated fats

There are two main groups of polyunsaturated fats: omega-6 and omega-3 polyunsaturates. The omega-6 fats tend to lower cholesterol, and these are found in safflower, sunflower and corn oils, and margarine made from these. The omega-3 fats also lower blood cholesterol and blood triglycerides, and reduce the risk of blood clotting. Good sources of omega-3 fats include fish, canola oil and margarine, and soybean oil.

How to Have Healthy Fats!

- Choose low-fat dairy foods such as low-fat milk, yoghurt, cheese and icecream.
- Replace saturated fats with unsaturated fats and carbohydrate-rich foods, e.g. use olive oil or canola oil instead of solid cooking fats, and spread honey, jam or avocado on your bread instead of butter or margarine.
- Choose lean meat and poultry, removing the skin and any visible fat. Avoid luncheon meats, salami and fatty sausages, and enjoy plenty of fish.
- Avoid fried and baked take away foods like chips, pies, pastries, cakes, biscuits and cookies that are high in fat.

In addition to reducing your fat intake, follow these strategies for reducing your risk of heart disease:

- Maintain a healthy weight.
- Increase your soluble fibre intake by eating more legumes, such as baked beans, chick peas and lentils, as well as oats, rice, barley and their brans, and fresh fruit and vegetables.
- Eat more soya-bean products, such as soy drinks, tofu, tempeh, soy flour and, of course, soy beans.
- Eat more fruit and vegetables, as these are good sources of antioxidants as well as fibre.
- Eat five or six small meals a day rather than two or three large ones. 'Grazing' (eating small amounts of food throughout the day) is better for weight control, energy levels and cholesterol control.

Check Your Pulse

Tasty, cheap and highly regarded nutritionally, dried beans should not be viewed as merely the poor man's meat. They can be teamed with salads, meats and soups. They are available in packs or cans from supermarkets, try including them in your weekly menu.

- **Split peas** that are red in colour do not need to be soaked. Gently cooked with water they make a puree in around 20 minutes. Mix with a little margarine, and serve with other dishes. Green or yellow split peas require presoaking, and make excellent soup or dhal.
- **Lentils** range in colour from orange to green and brown lentils. They do need soaking, and will cook in around 40 minutes. Cooked to a puree they make dhal, a side serving for Indian curries.
- **Kidney beans** (Mexican chilli beans) are familiar to Mexican food aficionados. They are named after their shape, and form the base of refried beans used to make tacos (page 131). The convenience of cans means that you can rev up a dip, or toss beans through a salad, or add them to a chilli sauce or soup.
- **Chick peas** have a nutty taste and a meaty texture — but, best of all, they do not cause flatulence! They are available in cans, and you can quickly make up a popular Middle Eastern dip called hommus to snack on at your leisure.

HANDY MAN HINTS

- *Pulses in packets will dry out with storage, and will take longer to cook. Store in a cool place, and use within a year. Soaking dried beans speeds up the cooking, so does precooking in the microwave oven on DEFROST (30%) for 40 minutes.*
- *Cook the beans thoroughly until tender; under-cooked beans cause indigestion.*
- *Refrigerate or freeze leftover cooked beans; they reheat well.*
- *Dhal can be made quickly in a microwave oven by combining 100 g red lentils, with 600 ml boiling water, a pinch each of chilli, ginger, turmeric and coriander powder. Cover, and cook on HIGH (100%) for 10 minutes, stirring once. If the lentils are not quite cooked, stir thoroughly, then cover, and cook on HIGH (100%) for a further 5 minutes. Season to taste, and serve. Dhal takes about one hour to cook conventionally, and needs constant stirring.*

Don't be afraid to use canned legumes or pulses such as baked beans. They only require heating, and are just as nutritious as their dried equivalents. Legumes are an excellent source of soluble fibre, which can help reduce blood-cholesterol levels. They are a useful source of iron and protein for vegetarians.

Few people have the time to soak dried pulses overnight before cooking them for two hours. Look for Quickpulse precooked pulses. This Australian-grown and packed range includes chick peas, whole brown lentils and red kidney beans; they are presoaked and ready to eat, and contain no added preservatives, additives, salt or sugar.

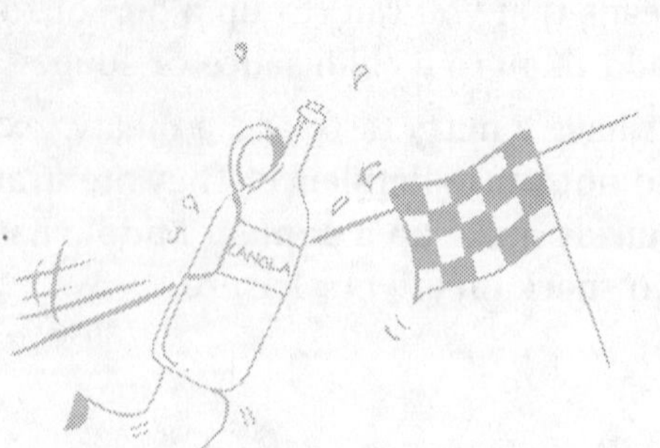

Par for the Course

Carbonara Chow Bella (page 115)
Green spinach salad with DIY Italian Dressing (page 149)
'Stoned' Dried-fruit Salad (page 164)

Fats take a long time to empty from your stomach, so it is important that the meal you eat before exercising is low in fats and oils. If you are using a small amount of oil in cooking or as a dressing or spread, choose one high in mono-unsaturates, e.g. canola oil or olive oil.

Laptop

Pizza Mushrooms (page 62)
Ricotta Ravioli Rocca (page 116)
Baked Apples with Attitude (page 161)

Fresh pastas are the best things to hit the supermarkets since sliced bread. A great source of carbohydrate and low in fat, they take ten minutes to prepare, and can be combined with fresh tomatoes, basil and other nutritious toppings and sauces. Always check the label of commercial sauces, and look for ones that do not use cream, cheese, butter or a lot of oil.

Italian Notebook

Macho Minestrone (page 55)
Pizza — A Slice of the Action (page 117)
Dating Game (page 195)

Legumes (such as red kidney beans) are rich in soluble fibre, which can help lower blood-cholesterol levels. Canned legumes are convenient and nutritious, and fabulous in soups and salads (see pages 109–10).

Add a glass of red wine, which is also believed to be beneficial in the fight against heart disease (but strictly in moderation!), and you have a delicious Mediterranean meal.

Older and Wiser

One-pot Chicken and Rice (page 118)
Steamed greens (page 52)
Blueberry and Mango Tango (page 192)

Each day aim to include rich red/orange-coloured fruits and vegetables like mango, cantaloupe, paw paw, peppers, carrot and pumpkin, in your meals, as they are good sources of vitamin A and C, both potent antioxidants that help in the fight against heart disease and cancer.

How to Cook Pasta

SERVES 2–4

8 cups water (conventional method); 5–6 cups hot water (microwave)
250 g slender pasta (spaghetti, linguini, penne, bows, bucatini, etc.)
1–2 tsp oil

CONVENTIONAL (15 MINUTES)

1 COOK according to the directions on the packet.
2 DRAIN, and use immediately. Remember that fresh pasta cooks a little more quickly.

large saucepan
teaspoon
cup measure
colander

MICROWAVE (15 MINUTES)

1 PLACE the water in the microwave-safe jug. Cover, and cook on HIGH (100%) for 6–7 minutes to bring to the boil. Add the oil and pasta.
2 PARTIALLY cover with plastic wrap, and cook on HIGH (100%) for 7–9 minutes, stirring several times during the cooking time.
3 DRAIN, and use immediately.

cup measure
teaspoon
large microwave-safe glass jug
plastic wrap
colander

To reheat pasta: Place the cooked pasta in a colander, and cover. Steam over a saucepan with a little boiling water until the pasta is heated through.

HANDY MAN HINTS

- *Pasta must be cooked in a large volume of boiling water, with 1 tbsp oil to prevent the pasta sticking together, and stirred.*
- *Cooking times vary with the different pastas, and fresh pastas cook more quickly than dried pastas. Well-cooked pasta will be firm or* al dente *(just tender).*
- *While I recommend specific pasta shapes in the recipes, you can use your own favourites, including wholemeal pasta.*
- *Use the microwave oven only when cooking small quantities of slender pasta.*
- *Immediately it is cooked, drain the pasta in a colander, then toss it in a bowl or saucepan with seasoning and sauce.*

How to Cook White Rice

Serves 3–4

1 cup white rice
1 tsp oil
1¾ cups lukewarm water

CONVENTIONAL (20 MINUTES)

1 USE the absorption method, according to the directions on the packet.

cup measure
teaspoon
large saucepan
colander
serving spoon

MICROWAVE (15 MINUTES)

1 PLACE the rice, oil and water in the microwave-safe container, and position it off the centre of the turntable.
2 COOK, uncovered, on HIGH (100%) for 10–12 minutes, until all the water is absorbed.
3 FLUFF up the rice with a fork. Cover with paper towel, and allow to stand for 3–4 minutes before serving.

cup measure
teaspoon
medium-sized microwave-safe container
fork
non-recycled paper towel
serving spoon

HANDY MAN HINTS

- *Use leftover rice to make fried rice, a salad or a pudding.*
- *Rice freezes well.*

VARIATION *Cook white rice in stock for extra flavour.*

How to Cook Brown Rice

Serves 3–4

1 cup brown rice
1 tsp oil
2 cups lukewarm water

CONVENTIONAL (30–38 MINUTES)

cup measure
teaspoon
large saucepan
serving spoon

1 USE the absorption method, according to the instructions on the packet.

MICROWAVE (25–30 MINUTES)

cup measure
teaspoon
medium-sized microwave-safe container, and lid
serving spoon

1 PLACE the rice, oil and water in the microwave-safe container. Cover and cook on HIGH (100%) for 5 minutes, then on MEDIUM (50–60%) for 20 minutes.
2 STIR the rice. Cover, and allow to stand for 3–5 minutes.

HANDY MAN HINT

The degree of rice tenderness is a preferred choice. Test a few grains — if the centre is still hard, continue cooking until the rice is tender.

Carbonara Chow Bella

Serves 2

560 g spaghetti, cooked
1 tbsp oil
1 large clove garlic, peeled and chopped
4 rashers rindless lean bacon, chopped
¼ cup white wine (or water)
1 (55 g) egg
½ cup grated Parmesan cheese or low-fat tasty cheese
black pepper, freshly ground, to taste

CONVENTIONAL (15 MINUTES)

1 COOK the pasta according to the directions on the packet, and drain. Keep the pasta warm.
2 COMBINE the oil, garlic and bacon in the frypan, and cook over high heat, stirring frequently, until they are soft and golden. Reduce the heat to low, add the wine or water, and simmer for 2 minutes.
3 ADD the cooked pasta, the egg and cheeses, and season with black pepper. Mix together evenly.

Serve immediately, with a spinach salad.

saucepan
colander
tablespoon
chopping board
small knife
cup measure
grater
non-stick frypan
egg lifter
serving spoon

MICROWAVE (10 MINUTES)

1 COOK the pasta in a large microwave-safe container according to the directions, on the packet, and drain. Keep the pasta warm.
2 HEAT the oil, garlic, bacon and white wine in the microwave-safe container on HIGH (100%) for 4 minutes.
3 STIR in the cooked pasta, the egg and cheese, and season with black pepper. Mix together evenly.

Serve immediately, with a spinach salad.

large microwave-safe container
colander
tablespoon
chopping board
small knife
cup measure
grater
spoon

HANDY MAN HINTS

- *To save time, cook the pasta on the stovetop while you make the sauce in the microwave.*
- *Yet another reason to eat your spinach! People who eat a lot of spinach have less macular degeneration (an age-related vision problem that is not fixed by wearing glasses).*

Ricotta Ravioli Rocca

Serves 2

8 cups cold water (conventional method); 5 cups hot water (microwave)
1 (635 g) packet fresh ricotta ravioli
1 tomato, chopped
2 tbsp pesto (page 152)
½ cup canned light evaporated milk
grated Parmesan cheese, for sprinkling (optional)
black pepper, freshly ground, to taste

CONVENTIONAL (25 MINUTES)

chopping board
knife
tablespoon
can opener
cup measure
large saucepan
colander
wooden spoon

1 PLACE the water in the saucepan, and bring to the boil. Add the ravioli. Cook according to the directions on the packet. Drain, and keep warm.
2 COMBINE the tomato and pesto in the saucepan, and cook over low heat for 4–5 minutes, stirring all the time. Add the milk, and cook for a further 2 minutes or until warmed through.
3 RETURN the pasta to the saucepan, and toss with the warm sauce.

Season with the cheese and pepper, and serve.

MICROWAVE (20 MINUTES)

chopping board
knife
tablespoon
can opener
cup measure
large microwave-safe container
colander
spoon

1 PLACE the hot water in the microwave-safe container. Cover, and cook on HIGH (100%) for 8 minutes. Add the ravioli, and cook on HIGH (100%) for 8 minutes. Drain, and keep warm.
2 COMBINE the pesto and tomato in the microwave-safe container, and cook on HIGH (100%) for 1 minute. Add the milk, and cook on HIGH (100%) for a further 2 minutes.
3 RETURN the pasta to the container, and toss with the warm sauce.

Season with the cheese and pepper, and serve.

HANDY MAN HINT *For a speedy meal, cook the ravioli on the stovetop, and at the same time cook the sauce in a microwave oven.*

VARIATION *Add 2 tbsp parsley or coriander.*

Pizza — a Slice of the Action

Serves 1–2

2 small pita pockets
1 tbsp tomato pasta sauce
1 (125 g) can smoked tuna slices, drained
1 tbsp shredded Parmesan cheese
1 tbsp reduced-fat mozzarella cheese
2 tbsp crumbled feta cheese

CONVENTIONAL (10–15 MINUTES)

Preheat the oven to 220°C.

1 LAYER each pita with the pasta sauce, tuna slices, and the three cheeses.
2 PLACE the prepared pizza on the baking tray, and bake for 5–10 minutes, or until the base is crispy and the cheese is melted.

Serve with a green salad and DIY Dressing (page 149).

tablespoon
can opener
metal baking tray

MICROWAVE (5 MINUTES)

1 LAYER each pita with the pasta sauce, tuna slices, and the three cheeses.
2 PLACE the prepared pizza on an upside-down dinner plate. Cover with paper towel, and cook on HIGH (100%) for 1–1½ minutes.

Serve with a green salad and DIY Dressing (page 149).

tablespoon
can opener
microwave-safe dinner plate
non-recycled paper towel

HANDY MAN HINTS

- *To crisp pita bread in the microwave oven, place it on a clean turntable, and cook, uncovered, on HIGH (100%) for 1½–2 minutes, turning the pita over halfway through the cooking time.*
- *A microwave roasting rack will help keep pizzas crisp.*

One-pot Chicken and Rice

Serves 2

2 tbsp olive oil
1 small onion, chopped
1 cup short-grain white rice
½ cup frozen peas
1 pkt Real Chicken Stock
1 cup water
500 g skinless chicken fillet, finely sliced
2 tbsp grated Parmesan cheese

CONVENTIONAL (35 MINUTES)

tablespoon
chopping board
knife
cup measure
grater
large saucepan, and lid
wooden spoon

1 HEAT the oil in the saucepan, and add the onion, rice and peas. Stir over medium heat for 3 minutes.
2 ADD the chicken stock and water. Cover, and simmer over low heat for 15 minutes, stirring occasionally.
3 STIR in the sliced chicken. Cover, and simmer for a further 10 minutes.

Serve with the Parmesan cheese sprinkled on top.

MICROWAVE (25 MINUTES)

tablespoon
chopping board
knife
cup measure
grater
large microwave-safe container, and lid
spoon

1 PLACE the onions, peas, rice and oil in the microwave-safe container. Cook, uncovered on HIGH (100%) for 4 minutes, stirring halfway through the cooking time.
2 ADD the chicken stock and water. Cover, and cook on HIGH (100%) for 10 minutes, stirring halfway through the cooking time.
3 STIR in the sliced chicken. Cover, and cook on HIGH (100%) for a further 5 minutes.

Serve with the Parmesan cheese sprinkled on top.

HANDY MAN HINT

Heat the stock and water before making this dish in the microwave oven, as it will shorten the cooking time.

FIT TIP

To boost your athletic performance, eat a meal rich in carbohydrates a couple of hours before exercising. Your body gets energy from the glucose released in your bloodstream through the digestion of carbohydrates.

ASIAN INSPIRATION

'With few exceptions, if it can't be cooked in minutes I don't want to know about it'

— Iain Hewitson.

And so say all of us, as most people do not want to spend hours shopping, chopping and cooking. Asian food offers an endless variety of tastes and flavours, and dishes are designed to be shared. Furthermore, Asian food caters from the budget blues to those who can afford banquet foods.

We can learn a lot about good nutrition from cultures around the world. Many Asian dishes are based on healthy ingredients like grains, soy products and fresh vegetables and nuts. However, you do need to beware of the 'Westernised' Chinese-style take away dishes that are high in fat and salt. Prepare your favourite Chinese, Malaysian, Vietnamese and Thai meals with plenty of spices and seasonings, but go easy on the oil and high-salt ingredients.

Chow Down

BBQ Chicken Fried Rice (page 121)
San Choy Bow (Lettuce Parcels) (page 122)
Pleasures of the Flesh (page 198)

Green leafy vegetables, such as bok choy, spinach, broccoli, etc., are good sources of iron and folate. Iron is absorbed better from these vegetables if you combine them with another food rich in vitamin C (e.g. orange, fruit salad, peppers, tomato).

Use Your Noodle

Nik Nok Noodles (page 123)
Dating Game (page 195)

Noodles are made from a combination of flour, water and salt. Some noodles are fried before being dried and packaged, and are much higher in fat than those that are simply dried.

No-fuss Noodles with Lamb (page 124)
Fruit 'n' Nut Platter (page 194)

This must be one of the fastest and healthiest dinner party menus around. You'll stun your guests without stressing yourself.

Hokkien Noodles (page 43)
Low-fat icecream, with Purple or Golden Passionfruit (page 198)

Hokkien Noodles are generally low in fat, make a great high-carbo base for a quick recovery meal or even a salad, and are popular with kids.

Orient Express

'Give 'em Curry' Laksa (page 125)
Pappadums the Healthy Way (page 125)
Chilled Lychees and Honeydew Melon 'Bytes' (page 193)

Curries and chillies are believed to be great for boosting your metabolism, and that having hot foods first thing in the morning has the best effect. However, chilli-flavoured breakfast cereal has yet to hit the market!

Hong Kong Kofta

Short Soup (page 126)
Asian Kofta Burgers (page 127)
Jellied fruit (page 165, variations) **and low-fat ice cream**

Look for low-salt varieties of stock cubes, soup stocks, soy sauce and other seasonings. MSG (monosodium glutamate) is high in sodium (the undesirable part of salt) too. Your taste for salt adjusts with time, so if you are a heavy salt user gradually reduce your intake, rather than going 'cold turkey'.

BBQ Chicken Fried Rice

SERVES 2

250 g skinless BBQ chicken, shredded
100 g broccoli florets
4 spring onions, chopped
2 tbsp BBQ sauce
2½ cups cooked rice (pages 113, 114), at room temperature

CONVENTIONAL (10 MINUTES)

1 HEAT a non-stick frypan over medium heat. Add the chicken, broccoli, onions and BBQ sauce, stirring thoroughly to combine.
2 COOK over medium heat for 3–4 minutes. Add the rice, stirring to mix together.
3 COOK for a further 3 minutes to heat the rice through.

Serve with a garnish of shredded spinach or lettuce leaves.

chopping board
knife
scales
tablespoon
cup measure
non-stick frypan
wooden spoon

MICROWAVE (8 MINUTES)

1 COMBINE the chicken, broccoli, onions and BBQ sauce in the microwave-safe container, stirring thoroughly to combine.
2 COVER, and cook on HIGH (100%) for 4 minutes, stirring halfway through the cooking time.
3 ADD the rice, stirring to mix together. Cover, and cook on HIGH (100%) for 2 minutes.

Serve with a garnish of shredded spinach or lettuce leaves.

chopping board
knife
scales
tablespoon
cup measure
large microwave-safe container, and lid
spoon

HANDY MAN HINT

Ready-washed salad leaves are now available at local supermarkets (page 86).

San Choy Bow (Lettuce Parcels)

SERVES 2

1 tbsp light soy sauce
1 tbsp plum sauce
1 tbsp light oil
250 g lean pork mince
1 clove garlic, crushed
4 spring onions, sliced diagonally
4 lettuce cups, chilled

CONVENTIONAL (10 MINUTES)

1 MIX together the soy and plum sauces in a small jug. Heat the oil in a wok over high heat for 30 seconds, and stir-fry the pork and garlic for 4 minutes.
2 ADD the spring onions and sauces, and cook over high heat for 1½ minutes.

Serve in the lettuce cups.

tablespoon
scales
chopping board
knife
small jug
spoon
wok
wooden spoon

MICROWAVE (10 MINUTES)

1 MIX together the soy and plum sauces in a small jug. Add the oil to the microwave-safe container. Cook, uncovered, on HIGH (100%) for 30 seconds.
2 STIR in the pork and garlic. Cook, uncovered, on HIGH (100%) for 3–4 minutes, stirring halfway through the cooking time.
3 ADD the spring onions and sauces. Cook, uncovered, on HIGH (100%) for 1½ minutes.

Serve in the lettuce cups.

tablespoon
scales
chopping board
knife
small jug
spoon
medium-sized microwave-safe container

HANDY MAN HINT *Finely ground lean mince produces the best results in microwave cooking, and is a healthier option.*

VARIATION *Add a can of drained and sliced water chestnuts to the pork stir-fry at step 3.*

Nik Nok Noodles

Serves 2

1 tbsp oil
½ red pepper, thinly sliced
1 cup broccoli florets
100 g mushrooms, thinly sliced
4 spring onions, chopped
4 pkts 2-minute Oriental noodle cakes (including seasoning)
4 cups hot water

CONVENTIONAL (15 MINUTES)

tablespoon
chopping board
knife
cup measure
large saucepan, and lid
wooden spoon

1 HEAT the oil in the saucepan over medium heat for 1 minute. Add the vegetables, and cook for a further 5 minutes, stirring once halfway through the cooking time.
2 CRUSH the noodle cakes, and add to the vegetables, plus the contents of two sachets of seasoning, and mix together evenly.
3 ADD the hot water, and stir. Cover, and cook on medium heat for 4 minutes.

Serve with shredded bok choy leaves.

MICROWAVE (12–15 MINUTES)

tablespoon
chopping board
knife
cup measure
large microwave-safe container, and lid
spoon

1 COMBINE the oil and vegetables in the microwave-safe container. Cook, uncovered, on HIGH (100%) for 2 minutes.
2 CRUSH the noodle cakes, and add to the vegetables, plus the contents of two sachets of seasoning, and mix together evenly.
3 ADD the hot water. Cover, and cook on HIGH (100%) for 4–6 minutes.

Serve with shredded bok choy leaves.

HANDY MAN HINTS

- *For speedy and convenient cooking, crush the noodle cakes in the bag before opening.*
- *Use a microwave oven if the weather is hot — you and your kitchen will stay cool.*

No-fuss Noodles with Lamb

SERVES 2

250 g lean lamb stir-fry strips
2 tbsp salt-reduced soy sauce
1 tsp sugar
3 spring onions, chopped diagonally
1 (375 g) pkt liquid chicken stock
1 (500 g) pkt noodles (or fresh Hokkien egg noodles)
1 cup hot water

CONVENTIONAL (15 MINUTES)

1 COMBINE the lamb, soy sauce, sugar and onions in the saucepan. Cook over high heat for 3–4 minutes, stirring regularly.
2 ADD the chicken stock, noodles and water, and stir. Cover, and cook over high heat for 5–6 minutes to bring to the boil.

Serve in soup bowls.

scales
tablespoon
teaspoon
chopping board
knife
cup measure
large saucepan, and lid
soup ladle

MICROWAVE (10 MINUTES)

1 COMBINE the lamb, soy sauce, sugar and onions in the microwave-safe container. Cook, uncovered, on HIGH (100%) for 2 minutes.
2 ADD the chicken stock, noodles and water, and stir. Cover, and cook on HIGH (100%) for 5 minutes.

Serve in soup bowls.

scales
tablespoon
teaspoon
chopping board
knife
cup measure
large microwave-safe container, and lid
spoon
soup ladle

HANDY MAN HINT *Tender lamb fillets are the best cut to use for stir-fries.*

VARIATION *Any selections of green vegetables may be added, e.g. spinach leaves, bean shoots or bok choy.*

'Give 'em Curry' Laksa

SERVES 2

2 small (100 g) bundles rice vermicelli
boiling water to cover
100 g celery, sliced diagonally
1 tsp green curry paste
1 (375 g) pkt liquid chicken stock
½ cup hot water
250 g BBQ chicken (skin removed), shredded
100 g bean shoots

CONVENTIONAL (15 MINUTES)

cup measure
scales
chopping board
knife
teaspoon
shallow dish
colander
large saucepan, and lid
spoon
soup ladle

1 PLACE the vermicelli in the shallow dish, and pour the boiling water over. Allow to stand for 2 minutes, then drain.
2 COMBINE the celery and curry paste in the saucepan, and cook over low heat for 1 minute, stirring occasionally. Pour in the chicken stock and ½ cup water. Add the vermicelli, and cook over high heat for 4–5 minutes. Add the chicken and bean shoots, and stir through.
3 COVER, and allow to stand for 4 minutes.

*Serve in large soup bowls, with **Pappadums** (page 126).*

MICROWAVE (12 MINUTES)

cup measure
scales
chopping board
teaspoon
shallow dish
colander
large microwave-safe container, and lid
spoon
soup ladle

1 PLACE the vermicelli in a shallow dish, and pour the boiling water over. Allow to stand for 2 minutes, then drain.
2 COMBINE the celery and curry paste in the microwave-safe container. Cook, uncovered, on HIGH (100%) for 1 minute. Pour in the chicken stock and ½ cup water. Add vermicelli. Cover, and cook on HIGH (100%) for 4–5 minutes. Add the chicken and bean shoots, and stir through.
3 COVER, and allow to stand for 4 minutes.

*Serve in large soup bowls, with **Pappadums** (page 126).*

HANDY MAN HINT

Vermicelli is made from the dough of finely-ground rice flour, and is readily available in supermarkets. It is quick and easy to use, and can be mixed with a variety of ingredients, such as seafood or vegetables.

Pappadums the Healthy Way

3 pappadums

MICROWAVE (1 MINUTE)

1 PLACE the pappadums on the outer rim of the turntable. Cook, uncovered on HIGH (100%) for 1 minute.

Note: 5 pappadums take 1½ minutes.

Serve with 'Give 'em Curry' Laksa (page 125).

Short Soup

SERVES 2

1 (375 g) pkt liquid chicken stock
2 cups (500 ml) hot water
4 chicken wings
2 spring onions, sliced diagonally
6 frozen wontons

CONVENTIONAL (45 MINUTES)

1 PLACE the chicken stock, water and chicken wings in the saucepan, and bring to the boil over high heat (about 10 minutes).
2 COVER the pan, and simmer the soup over very low heat for 25 minutes.
3 REMOVE the chicken wings, and add the onions and wontons. Leave uncovered, and simmer for a further 5 minutes.

Serve in Chinese soup bowls.

cup measure
chopping board
knife
small saucepan, and lid
slotted spoon

MICROWAVE (22 MINUTES)

1 PLACE the chicken stock, water and chicken wings into the microwave-safe jug. Cover, and cook on HIGH (100%) for 5 minutes.
2 COOK on MEDIUM (50–60%) for 10 minutes.
3 REMOVE the chicken wings, and add the onions and wontons. Cover, and cook on HIGH (100%) for a further 4 minutes.

Serve in Chinese soup bowls.

cup measure
chopping board
knife
microwave-safe jug
plastic wrap
slotted spoon

Asian Kofta Burgers

Serves 2

250 g lean beef mince
1 tbsp soy sauce
1 tbsp chilli sauce
1 tsp finely chopped fresh coriander
2 spring onions, chopped
4 burger buns (split)
mixed lettuce leaves

CONVENTIONAL (15 MINUTES)

1 COMBINE all the ingredients, except the buns and lettuce, in the bowl. When the mixture is evenly combined, shape it into four oval-shaped burgers.

2 HEAT the frypan over medium heat, add the burgers, and cook for 6 minutes, turning them over halfway through the cooking time.

Place lettuce leaves and a burger inside each bun to serve.

scales
tablespoon
chopping board
knife
bread knife
mixing bowl
spoon
non-stick frypan
egg lifter

MICROWAVE (10 MINUTES)

1 COMBINE all the ingredients, except the buns and lettuce, in the bowl. When the mixture is evenly combined, shape it into four oval-shaped burgers.

2 PLACE two sheets of paper towel on an upturned dinner plate, and put the burgers on top. Cover with two sheets of paper towel, and cook on HIGH (100%) for 4 minutes.

Place lettuce leaves and a burger inside each bun to serve.

scales
tablespoon
chopping board
knife
bread knife
mixing bowl
spoon
microwave-safe dinner plate
non-recycled paper towel

HANDY MAN HINT

Once cooked, the burgers will freeze successfully.

Hot to Trot

Chilli Peppers

Sweet, mild or pungent chillies are popular ingredients in our kitchens. As a rule, the smaller the chilli, the bigger the kick. The Aussie rule is less is more!

Heat rating for hard-core chilli-heads:1 chilli, mild; 2 chillies, medium; 3 chillies, hot; 4 chillies, very hot.

Anaheim: mild to medium, green, with a sweet flavour, and about 15 cm long. Add to Italian- and Spanish-style foods.

Jalapeno: hot to very hot, green, with a thick skin, about 5 cm long. Use in tacos, tortillas, salsas and dips.

Thai: fiery little devils, purple, red or orange, about 1.5 cm long. Add to laksa, salsa or stir-fries.

Safety

- Wash your hands thoroughly after handling chillies.
- Do not rub your eyes after preparing chillies.

First aid: Wash your hands thoroughly, then splash your eyes with plenty of cold water.

Curry in a Hurry

Try these flavours, all readily available in bottles, cans or packs.

Thai green curry is distinguished by the use of coriander and coconut milk, mixed with other ingredients for an exotic flavour.

Thai red curry is a stronger version than green curry for meat, chicken or fish.

Madras curry is a spicy introduction to curry from southern India, it is prepared with chilli and coconut, and is good for lamb curries.

Tandoori paste is a marinade for chicken and lamb, and is made with spices such as paprika, coriander, cumin and ginger, mixed with yoghurt. It is good for barbecues and grills.

Vindaloo curry is a hot, pungent and fragrant Indian curry paste; it makes a good beef curry that improves over a few days.

Satay sauce is a spicy blend from Indonesia. It combines peanut butter, coconut milk and other spices. Brush it over chicken, prawns or meat on skewers before cooking.

BEERS WITH THE BOYS

'Macho does not prove mucho'

— Zsa Zsa Gabor.

Inebriation is not 'in' any more, so if you are having a drink make sure you also have high-carbo snacks and non-alcoholic drinks to accompany the beer. This way you will not only please the police, but your partner too — and your head the next day!

FIT TIPS Alcohol — the good, the bad and the ugly. The good news is that low-risk drinking of an average of one or two standard drinks a day may well be beneficial to your health. The bad news is that excessive drinking is definitely bad for your health, and may contribute to impotence! Work and sports performance are also likely to be adversely affected by alcohol. The ugly — well, we've probably all seen ourselves or our mates after a few too many.

So if you enjoy a beer with the boys, or a wine with the wife, make sure it is in moderation, and watch what is being washed down with the alcohol. Typical pub fare is high in fat and very high in salt (to encourage you to drink more), and alcohol makes you particularly hungry! Instead of picking up takeaways, try some of these easy, quick alternatives.

Short-order Chef

Nuts to crack

Punters' Popcorn

Serves 2

¼ cup popping corn
1 tsp water

MICROWAVE (5 MINUTES)

cup measure
teaspoon
oven bag
rubber band

1. PLACE the corn in an oven bag. Sprinkle with water.
2. SECURE the bag with a rubber band, and cook on HIGH (100%) for 4 minutes, turning the bag over halfway through the cooking time.

HANDY MAN HINT

Do not overload the oven bag with uncooked corn, as it will not cook properly.

One-for-the-road Taco

SERVES 2

300 g lean beef mince
1 tbsp taco seasoning
1 (450 g) can Mexican Chilli beans
lettuce leaves
¼ cup taco sauce
¼ cup grated low-fat cheese
6 taco shells (warmed)

CONVENTIONAL (12 MINUTES)

1 BROWN the mince in the frypan over high heat for 5 minutes, stirring regularly. Add taco seasoning, mixing through evenly.
2 STIR in the beans. Cook over medium heat for 3–4 minutes to warm through.

Place the lettuce, beef and bean mix, taco sauce and cheese in warmed taco shells to serve.

scales
tablespoon
can opener
spoon
cup measure
non-stick frypan
wooden spoon

MICROWAVE (10 MINUTES)

1 CRUMBLE the mince into the microwave-safe container. Cook, uncovered, on HIGH (100%) for 3–4 minutes, then drain off any excess liquid. Stir in the taco seasoning, mixing through evenly.
2 STIR in the beans. Cover, and cook on HIGH (100%) for 2–3 minutes to warm through.

Place the lettuce, beef and bean mix, taco sauce and cheese in warmed taco shells to serve.

scales
tablespoon
can opener
spoon
cup measure
large microwave-safe container and lid

HANDY MAN HINT *You can easily heat six taco shells in the microwave; cook on HIGH (100%) for 1 minute.*

FIT TIP *Refried beans are low in fat, high in protein and a great source of fibre.*

Souvlaki Takeaway

SERVES 2

1 tsp olive oil
2 large pita breads
300 g lean beef, cubed
2 mushrooms, sliced
lettuce leaves
1 tomato, sliced
tomato sauce or tzatiki dip

teaspoon
scales
chopping board
knife
spoon

CONVENTIONAL (15 MINUTES)

1 HEAT the oil in the frypan over medium heat for 30 seconds, and brown each pita bread on each side for 30 seconds.
2 REMOVE the bread, and add the meat. Cook over medium heat for 8 minutes, stirring halfway through the cooking time.
3 ASSEMBLE the souvlaki: place the pita bread on a flat surface and cover with lettuce, mushrooms, tomato, tomato sauce or tzatiki dip, and finish with the meat.

Roll up, and serve.

HANDY MAN HINT *Place the filling on one half of the pita bread for easier rolling.*

VARIATION *Use Tomato Sauce Supreme (page 151) instead of tomato sauce.*

Short-pass Savoury Cheese Squares

SERVES 2

1 puff pastry sheet
1 tbsp chutney of your choice
1 (225 g) can pineapple pieces, well drained
1 cup shredded BBQ chicken, skin removed (optional)
1½ cups grated low-fat tasty cheese

CONVENTIONAL (25–30 MINUTES)

Preheat the oven to 200°C.

1 PLACE the pastry sheet on the baking tray. Spread the chutney evenly over the pastry sheet, and cut the sheet into four squares.
2 TOP each square with the remaining ingredients, finishing with the cheese on top.
3 BAKE for 15–25 minutes until the surface is golden and crisp.

Serve with a salad.

chopping board
knife
tablespoon
can opener
spoon
cup measure
metal baking tray
table knife

VARIATIONS *Try toppings such as lean ham, sliced mushrooms, or sweetcorn kernels.*

Chilli Hot Dogs

SERVES 2

2 cups water (conventional method only)
2 hot dog frankfurts, pierced three times with a fork
2 slices Swiss-style cheese
2 hot dog rolls, split
2 tbsp mustard of your choice
mixed lettuce leaves
1 (130 g) can baked beans (optional)
1 tbsp chilli sauce

CONVENTIONAL (15 MINUTES)

fork
bread knife
tablespoon
can opener
spoon
medium-sized saucepan
colander
table knife

1 PLACE the water in the saucepan and bring to the boil. Add the frankfurts, and cook over medium heat for 5–8 minutes. Drain off the water.
2 SPREAD the mustard over the bottom half of each roll, and layer the lettuce leaves, cheese, hot dogs and baked beans; top with the chilli sauce.
3 COVER with the top half of the roll.

Serve immediately.

MICROWAVE (5–6 MINUTES)

fork
bread knife
tablespoon
can opener
spoon
table knife
non-recycled paper towel

1 PLACE the frankfurts on the edge of the turntable. Cook, uncovered, on HIGH (100%) for 40 seconds.
2 SPREAD the mustard over the bottom half of each roll, and layer the lettuce leaves, cheese, hot dogs and baked beans; top with the chilli sauce.
3 COVER with the top half of the roll. Wrap each roll in paper towel, and reheat each roll on HIGH (100%) for 30 seconds. Remove the paper towel.

Serve immediately.

VARIATIONS *Try more adventurous toppings, such as canned asparagus, pickles, pesto, sweetcorn kernels, peanut sauce or taco sauce.*

Pizza Mexican Style

SERVES 2

2 small snack pitas (5 cm oval pockets)
½ tbsp taco sauce
½ tbsp chilli sauce
½ red pepper, sliced
60 g low-fat hot salami, sliced
40 g low-fat mozzarella cheese, grated

CONVENTIONAL (10–15 MINUTES)

Preheat the oven to 220°C.

1 COMBINE the taco and chilli sauces, and spread each pita bread with this mixture. Top with the pepper, salami, and cheese.
2 PLACE the pizzas on the baking tray, and bake for 5–10 minutes, or until the base is crisp and the cheese has melted.

Serve with Mexican Salsa (page 153).

tablespoon
chopping board
knife
grater
metal baking tray

MICROWAVE (5 MINUTES)

1 COMBINE the taco and chilli sauces, and spread each pita bread with this mixture. Top with the pepper, salami, and cheese.
2 PLACE paper towel on an upside-down dinner plate, and put the pizzas on top. Cook on HIGH (100%) for 1 minute.

Serve with Mexican Salsa (page 153).

tablespoon
chopping board
knife
grater
microwave-safe dinner plate
non-recycled paper towel

HANDY MAN HINT

To remove excess fat before adding to the pizza, place the slices of salami on paper towel on the microwave turntable, and cook on HIGH (100%) for 1 minute.

VARIATION

Use lean ham (such as Virginia or gypsy ham) in place of salami for a lower fat option.

Pita Chips

4 small pita rounds

SERVES 1

CONVENTIONAL (10–12 MINUTES)

knife
metal baking tray

Preheat the oven to 200°C.

1 PULL or cut two pita rounds apart.
2 PLACE the rounds on the baking tray, and bake for 5–10 minutes until crisp.
3 ALLOW to stand until cool, then break the rounds into small pieces.
Repeat the procedure for the remaining pitas.

Serve with Chick Pea and Garlic Dip (page 137), or dips of your choice.

MICROWAVE (4 MINUTES)

knife

1 PULL or cut two pita rounds apart.
2 PLACE the rounds on the turntable. Cook, uncovered, on HIGH (100%) for 2 minutes.
3 ALLOW to stand until cool, then break the rounds into small pieces.

Repeat the procedure for the remaining pitas.

Serve with Chick Pea and Garlic Dip (page 137), Weight Watcher's Dip or Smoked Tuna Dip (page 138), Hommus Skinny Dip (page 184), or dips of your choice.

HANDY MAN HINT *Make sure your microwave turntable is clean. Greasy spills attract microwaves, and slow down your cooking time.*

VARIATIONS *Brush pita rounds with olive oil or pesto, and sprinkle with Parmesan cheese or a spice of your choice, before cooking.*

Chick Pea and Garlic Dip

SERVES 2

1 (130 g) can chick peas, drained
2 cloves garlic, peeled
juice of ½ lemon
½ cup natural or plain yoghurt
½ tsp dried or chopped fresh coriander

CONVENTIONAL (8 MINUTES)

1 PLACE all the ingredients in the blender, and blend in 1-minute bursts, stirring between.
2 BLEND for 4 minutes.

Serve with Pita Chips (page 136).

can opener
strainer
chopping board
knife
lemon juicer
cup measure
teaspoon
blender
spoon

HANDY MAN HINT

To peel 2 cloves of garlic quickly in a microwave oven, heat them on HIGH (100%) for 15–20 seconds. Squeeze at one end until the cloves pop out of the skins.

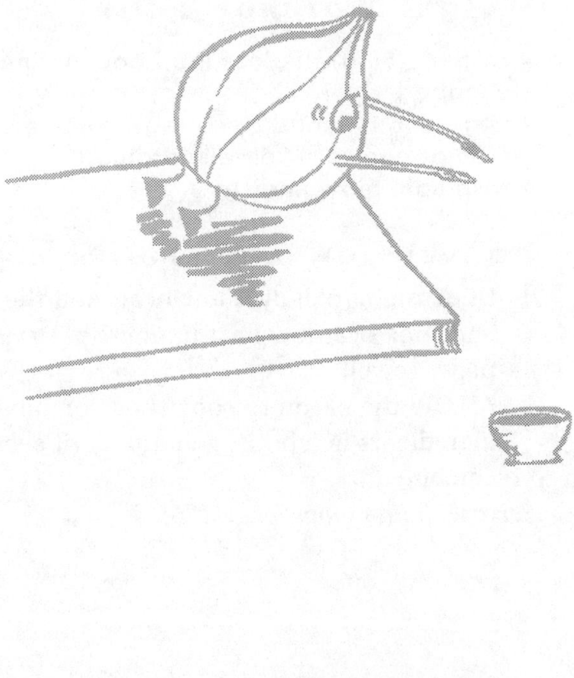

Smoked Tuna Dip

SERVES 4

100 g light cream cheese
1 (125 g) can smoked tuna, drained
20 g capers
40 g semi-sundried tomatoes, chopped
juice of ½ lemon
5 g chopped chives

CONVENTIONAL (5 MINUTES)

1 COMBINE all the ingredients in a bowl, mixing with a fork until evenly combined.

Serve with Pita Chips (page 136).

scales
can opener
spoon
chopping board
knife
lemon juicer
mixing bowl
fork

HANDY MAN HINT *Snip the chives with scissors.*

Weight Watcher's Dip

SERVES 2

4 rashers (80 g) rindless lean bacon, finely chopped
125 g smooth ricotta or cottage cheese
1 (150 g) can corn kernels, drained
1 tbsp light mayonnaise

CONVENTIONAL (8 MINUTES)

1 HEAT the frypan over low heat. Add the bacon, and cook over low heat until crisp. Drain on paper towel.
2 ALLOW the bacon to cool, then combine all the ingredients in a bowl, and mix until evenly combined.

Serve with Pita Chips (page 136).

chopping board
knife
scales
can opener
strainer
tablespoon
non-stick frypan
paper towel
mixing bowl
spoon or fork

Macaroni Cheese Masterpiece

Serves 2

water (as specified on pasta packet)
250 g macaroni (500 g cooked macaroni)
4 thin low-fat chicken sausages, pierced 6 times with a fork
1 cup white sauce } combined
1 tbsp tomato sauce } combined
½ cup grated low-fat tasty cheese

CONVENTIONAL (45 MINUTES)

Preheat the oven to 200°C.

fork
cup measure
grater
large saucepan
colander
non-stick frypan
ovenproof dish
spoon

1 PLACE the water in the saucepan and bring it to the boil. Add the pasta, and cook according to the directions on the packet. Drain.
2 COOK the sausages in the frypan over medium heat for 6 minutes. Transfer them to the ovenproof dish. Mix the cooked macaroni into the sauce, and spoon it over the sausages. Top with the cheese.
3 BAKE for 15 minutes, or until the cheese has browned.

Serve with coleslaw (page 79) and DIY Mustard Dressing (page 149).

MICROWAVE (30 MINUTES)

fork
cup measure
grater
large microwave-safe container, and lid
colander
spoon

1 PLACE the water in the microwave-safe container, and cook on HIGH (100%) for 10 minutes to bring it to the boil. Add the pasta, and cook according to the directions on the packet. Drain.
2 PLACE the sausages in the microwave-safe container. Cook, uncovered, on HIGH (100%) for 2 minutes. Mix the macaroni into the sauce, and spoon it over the sausages. Top with the cheese.
3 COVER, and cook on HIGH (100%) for 5 minutes.

Serve with coleslaw (page 79) and DIY Mustard Dressing (page 149).

HANDY MAN HINTS

- *Pasta takes about the same time to cook in a microwave oven as conventionally, because of the amount of water.*
- *Leftovers reheat well for lunch at work.*

FIT TIP *For the best perfomance, aim to eat a light low-fat meal or snack 2-3 hours before you exercise.*

VARIATION *Add ½ cup frozen peas or beans to make a meal-in-one.*

Low-fat Sandwich Login

These fillings are best spread on wholegrain bread or in wholegrain rolls.

- Banana, honey and ricotta.
- Light cream cheese, chopped dried apricots and pecan nuts.
- Your favourite light dip with lettuce and tomato.
- Cottage cheese with drained mixed beans and grated carrot.
- Celery with currants, pine nuts and grated carrot.
- Potato salad and cold BBQ chicken.
- Celery, cucumber, grated carrot, chopped walnuts and yoghurt.

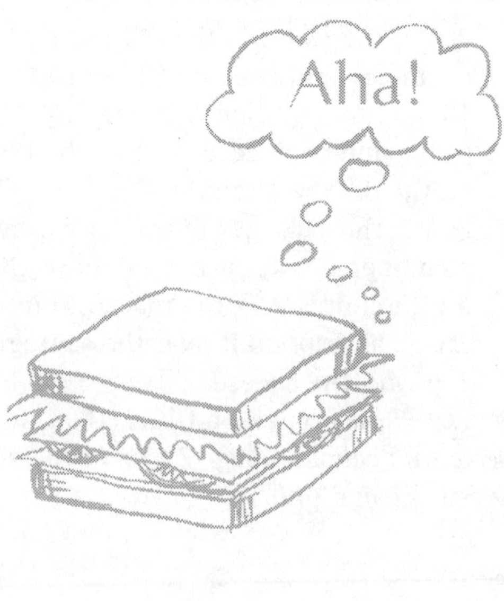

Kiss the Chef — Food and Your Sex Life

'The only people who should really sin are the people who can sin with a grin'

— Ogden Nash.

Kiss the chef, or whoever else you may feel like kissing at the time! Many foods have long been suggested as aphrodisiacs, and for other physical effects. Foods such as oysters, avocado, caviar and chocolate-dipped strawberries accompanied by chilled champagne, and the images they evoke — as well as the atmosphere they are consumed in — may be enough to send some couples off to the bedroom.

Fit Tips To be sexually healthy you need to be generally healthy, and a good diet is essential for health and fitness. If you are not in good shape, you are unlikely to be able to give a good performance in the bedroom! A couple of drinks may whet your sexual appetite, but excessive alcohol will decrease your libido — and put a dampener on your bedroom antics.

So, in addition to a high-carbohydrate, low-fat, varied diet, experiment with some of the suggested dishes, and see if they have any aphrodisiac properties for you!

Garlic — Aphrodisiac or Turn-off?

Like it or loathe it, garlic has long been considered an aphrodisiac, as well as having impressive medicinal claims such as lowering blood cholesterol, dilating arteries and treating intestinal disorders.

Gastronomically, garlic goes well with many foods, so here are some guidelines.

- When buying garlic, look for firm compact nobs, without any signs of sprouting or loose covering.
- Strong garlic flavours are achieved by smashing the garlic to release the essential oil. A light garlic flavour is achieved by peeling a clove, and chopping it finely to cook in a warm oil over a low heat. Garlic becomes milder the longer it cooks.
- Garlic odour clings to chopping boards and knives, to eliminate this, rub a cut lemon over them, then wash them well in cold water. Rub your hands with the cut lemon, then rinse them under cold water.
- To make garlic socially acceptable, make sure you and your dinner companion/s eat it at the same time. Chewing parsley or coffee beans may help remove traces of garlic odour. Copious quantities of garlic are not recommended for sales reps!

HANDY MAN HINT

To peel a garlic clove, place it on a chopping board, and put the flat part of a knife on top, and press down firmly. Or place a clove of garlic in a microwave oven, and cook on HIGH (100%) for 10 seconds; the skin will then slip off easily. Otherwise, use bottled garlic!

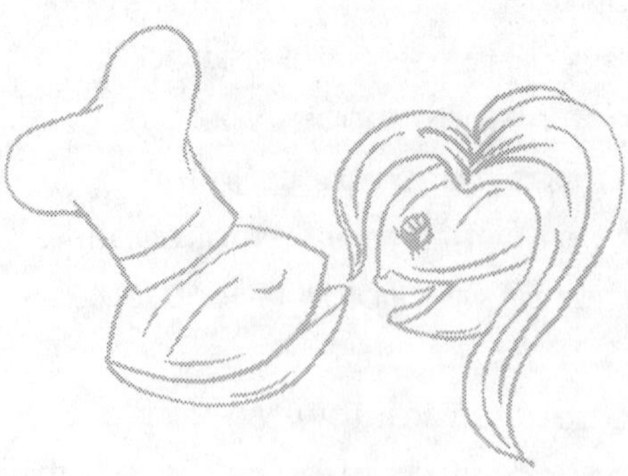

Delightfully Decadent

Mix 'n' match:

Gourmet Sandwiches (page 143)

Garlic Chilli Prawns (page 144)

Oysters Kilpatrick (page 145)

Crustless Egg and Bacon Pie (page 146)

Icecream Sundae Event (page 165)

Easy-as-apple Pie (page 158)

Masters' Cheesecake (page 167)

Dating Game (page 195)

Despite the fact that a healthy low-fat, high-carbohydrate eating plan is ideal for long-term health and fitness, psychological health is important too, and no dietitian would disagree that an indulgence now and then is good for the soul!

These dishes are truly indulgences, but enjoy them on special occasions — and don't feel guilty!

Gourmet Sandwiches

- Leftover chicken, with peanut butter and rocket.
- Smoked tuna or salmon, cream cheese, semi-dried tomatoes, on lettuce leaves.
- Camembert, dried fruit and mixed nuts.
- Avocado with lemon juice, prawns and lettuce mix.
- Horseradish, mixed with mayo, over sliced canned artichokes.

Garlic Chilli Prawns

SERVES 2

1 cup oil (conventional method); ¼ cup (microwave)
4 garlic cloves, peeled and finely chopped
1 small red chilli, chopped
500 g medium-sized green prawns (22–24), peeled and deveined
1 tbsp chopped parsley

CONVENTIONAL (7 MINUTES)

chopping board
knife
cup measure
tablespoon
non-stick frypan
wooden spoon

1 HEAT the oil in the frypan over medium heat for 1 minute, then add the garlic and chilli. Cook over high heat for 1 minute.
2 STIR in the prawns, and cook over high heat for 2 minutes, stirring constantly. Stir in the parsley.

Serve with lemon wedges over ***Hokkien Noodles*** *(page 43).*

MICROWAVE (7 MINUTES)

chopping board
knife
cup measure
tablespoon
large microwave-safe container
tongs

1 PLACE the oil in the microwave-safe container. Cook, uncovered, on HIGH (100%) for 1 minute. Then add the garlic and chilli, and cook, uncovered, on HIGH (100%) for 1 minute, stirring halfway through the cooking time.
2 ARRANGE the prawns on top with the tails pointing towards the centre. Cook, uncovered, on MEDIUM-HIGH (70–80%) for 3½ minutes, turning them over halfway through the cooking time. Stir in the parsley.

Serve with lemon wedges over ***Hokkien Noodles*** *(page 43).*

HANDY MAN HINT

To prepare prawns: peel off the shells, then make a slit down the back of each prawn, and remove the dark vein.

Oysters Kilpatrick

Serves 2

12 oysters in half-shells
3 tsp lemon juice
3 tsp Worcestershire sauce
1 lean rindless bacon rasher, finely chopped
black pepper, freshly ground, to taste

CONVENTIONAL (6–7 MINUTES)

teaspoon
lemon juicer
chopping board
knife
metal baking tray
serving tongs

1 PIERCE each oyster several times with a fork, and place the oysters in their shells on the baking tray.
2 THOROUGHLY combine the remaining ingredients, and add to the top of each oyster.
3 PLACE the tray under a preheated hot grill, and cook for 2–3 minutes, until the bacon is crispy.

Season with pepper, and serve with brown bread.

MICROWAVE (5 MINUTES)

teaspoon
lemon juicer
chopping board
knife
non-recycled paper towel
serving tongs

1 PIERCE each oyster several times with a fork. Place one sheet paper towel on a plain dinner plate, and put the oysters in their shells on top.
2 THOROUGHLY combine the remaining ingredients, and add to the top of each oyster. Cover with another sheet of paper towel.
3 COOK on HIGH (100%) for 1–2 minutes.

Season with pepper, and serve with brown bread.

HANDY MAN HINT

When choosing oysters in the half-shell, look for ones that are plump, creamy, glistening, and with a 'sea' smell. Reject oysters that look dull or have a strong smell.

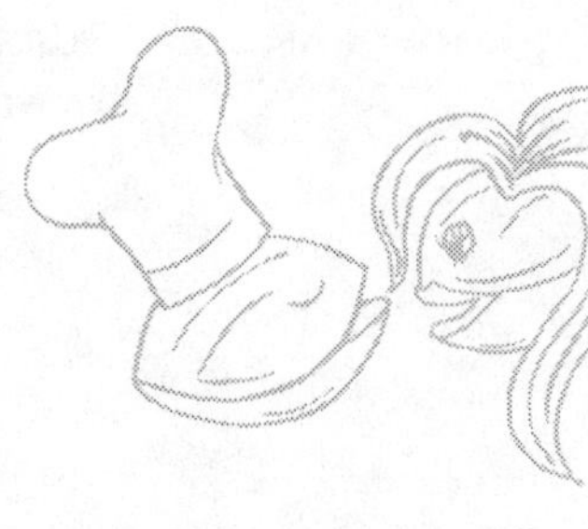

Crustless Egg and Bacon Pie

SERVES 2

1 small onion, chopped
4 rashers lean rindless bacon, cut into strips
4 (55 g) eggs, at room temperature
¼ cup milk, at room temperature
¼ cup low-fat grated tasty cheese
1 tbsp tomato sauce

CONVENTIONAL (20 MINUTES)

chopping board
knife
cup measure
grater
tablespoon
non-stick frypan, and lid
wooden spoon
mixing bowl
whisk or fork

1 PLACE the onion and bacon in the frypan, and cook over medium heat for 4 minutes.
2 WHISK together the eggs, milk, cheese and tomato sauce, and pour over the bacon mixture. Cover, and cook over low heat for 8–10 minutes until set.
3 ALLOW to stand for 1 minute, then slice.

Serve hot or cold, with wholegrain bread.

MICROWAVE (12 MINUTES)

chopping board
knife
cup measure
grater
tablespoon
medium-sized microwave-safe container
mixing bowl
whisk or fork
non-recycled paper towel

1 PLACE the onion and bacon in the microwave-safe container. Cook, uncovered, on HIGH (100%) for 3 minutes.
2 WHISK together the eggs, milk, cheese and tomato sauce, and pour over the bacon mixture. Cover loosely with paper towel, and cook on HIGH (100%) for 4–5 minutes.
3 ALLOW to stand for 1 minute for the centre to set, then slice.

Serve hot or cold, with wholegrain bread.

HANDY MAN HINT

Use pesto (page 152) instead of tomato sauce for a creative flavour.

Liquid Assets

'I don't know much about being a millionaire, but I'll bet I'd be a darling at it'

— Dorothy Parker.

No special cooking skills are required to rev up a simple savoury or sweet sauce that can make you seem a better cook than you may be.

For instance, if you're one of those shoppers I see regularly at the supermarket purchasing a mega-sized steak and smallish tomato for a meal, you can turn that tomato into a salsa. Salsa simply means sauce, either cooked or raw; salsas go well with fish, chicken, burgers or barbecued food. You merely need a cucumber, chilli flakes and a squeeze of lemon juice to provide dinner with a dash from readily available ingredients.

Sauces add culinary creativity to everyday food, and enhance your hero status inside and outside the kitchen.

Sauces and dressings can really make a dish — however, they should complement, not overpower. This means that you should add small amounts, particularly of those that are based on oil or other fats.

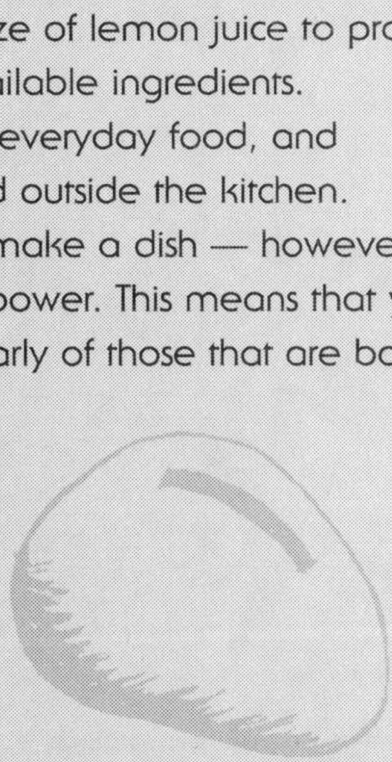

DIY Dressings

CONVENTIONAL (3 MINUTES)

SERVES 2

1 Dressings are easy to make, simply place all the ingredients in a clean screwtop jar, tighten the lid, and shake vigorously to blend.

Serve immediately.

- screwtop jar and lid
- cup measure
- tablespoon
- teaspoon
- lemon juicer
- chopping board
- knife

Italian

½ cup oil
2 tbsp vinegar
1 tbsp fresh basil (or dried)
½ tbsp oregano (optional)

Lemon

½ cup oil
2 tbsp lemon juice
1 clove garlic, peeled and chopped finely
black pepper, freshly ground, to taste

Mustard

½ cup oil
2 tbsp vinegar
2 tsp seeded mustard
salt and pepper, to taste

Orange and Honey

¾ cup orange juice
2 tbsp honey
2 tsp sesame seeds

Indian

½ cup oil
2 tbsp vinegar
1 tbsp coriander
1 tsp ginger powder
1 tsp chilli flakes (optional)

Rosemary

½ cup oil
2 tbsp lemon juice
1 tbsp rosemary, fresh or dried
1 clove garlic, finely chopped

Asian

⅓ cup oil
2 tbsp rice vinegar
1 tsp sesame seed oil
1 clove garlic, peeled and chopped finely

Lime and Yoghurt

2 tbsp light olive oil
2 tbsp fresh lime juice
1 level tbsp yoghurt
salt and pepper, to taste

HANDY MAN HINT

Good olive oil and balsamic vinegar are recommended to make an excellent tasting dressing.

White Sauce, Pure 'n' Simple

Makes 1 cup

25 g margarine
2 tbsp plain flour
1 cup low-fat milk, at room temperature
salt and pepper, to taste
¼ cup grated low-fat tasty cheese (optional)

CONVENTIONAL (7 MINUTES)

scales
tablespoon
cup measure
grater
small saucepan
wooden spoon

1 PLACE the margarine in the saucepan, and melt over a low heat. Remove from the heat, and stir in the flour, mixing evenly.
2 STIR over a low heat for 1–2 minutes to cook the flour, stir in a third of the milk until smooth, then add the remaining milk. Stir four times at 1-minute intervals, until smooth.
3 ADD the seasoning and cheese, stirring through evenly.

Serve immediately over vegetables or fish.

MICROWAVE (5 MINUTES)

scales
tablespoon
cup measure
grater
small microwave-safe container
spoon

1 PLACE the margarine in the base of the microwave-safe dish. Cook, uncovered, on HIGH (100%) for 30 seconds.
2 ADD the flour, and stir until evenly combined. Add a third of the milk, and stir well to dissolve. Blend in the remaining milk. Cook, uncovered, on HIGH (100%) for 3 minutes, stirring halfway through the cooking time.
3 ADD the seasoning and cheese, stirring through evenly.

Serve immediately over vegetables or fish.

HANDY MAN HINT

Full-fat milk is not necessary for making a good white sauce. Try some of the range of the low-fat milks for a healthier choice, as they are higher in calcium and protein.

VARIATION

For a sweet sauce, omit the salt and pepper, and the cheese, and stir in 1 tbsp sugar and 1 tsp vanilla essence towards the end of the cooking time.

Tomato Sauce Supreme

Enliven your favourite tomato sauce — to ½ cup tomato sauce add one of the following:

dash of seeded, chopped chillies
or 1 tbsp soy sauce
or 1 tbsp Worcestershire sauce
or 1–2 cloves crushed garlic
or 1 tsp curry seasoning
or 1 tsp lemon juice

CONVENTIONAL (3 MINUTES)

1 **MIX all the ingredients together, and store in a screwtop jar.**

Serve with steak or sausages.

chopping board
knife
tablespoon
teaspoon
lemon juicer
mixing bowl

HANDY MAN HINT

To bring tomato sauce to a pouring consistency, warm it in a microwave oven: remove the metal cap, and cook on HIGH (100%) for 30–60 seconds.

VARIATION

Add 1 tbsp pineapple pieces and 1 tbsp pineapple juice for a sweet 'n' sour sauce.

Pesto

Serves 2

1 bunch basil
60 g pine nuts
2 cloves garlic, peeled and crushed
60 g grated Parmesan cheese
½ cup olive oil

CONVENTIONAL (5 MINUTES)

chopping board
knife
scales
grater
cup measure
screwtop jar and lid

1 PLACE the basil, pine nuts, garlic and cheese in a blender or food processer, and blend to a paste.
2 ADD the oil, and blend until it is evenly combined.
3 USE immediately, or store in a sealed screwtop jar in the refrigerator for up to a month.

HANDY MAN HINT *Pesto is available bottled from the herb and spice section of supermarkets.*

VARIATION *This highly addictive sauce is good added to minestrone or pasta.*

Mango Salsa

Serves 2

1 slightly firm mango
1 small chilli, seeded and finely chopped
1½ tbsp lime or lemon juice
1 tbsp finely chopped spring onions
1 tbsp chopped fresh mint

CONVENTIONAL (5 MINUTES, PLUS STANDING TIME)

chopping board
knife
tablespoon
mixing bowl
spoon

1 CHOP the mango flesh into small dice, and place in the mixing bowl.
2 ADD the chilli, lime juice, onion and mint, and stir through.
3 PLACE this in the refrigerator for 1 hour to allow the flavours to develop.

Serve over grilled fish, prawns or chicken.

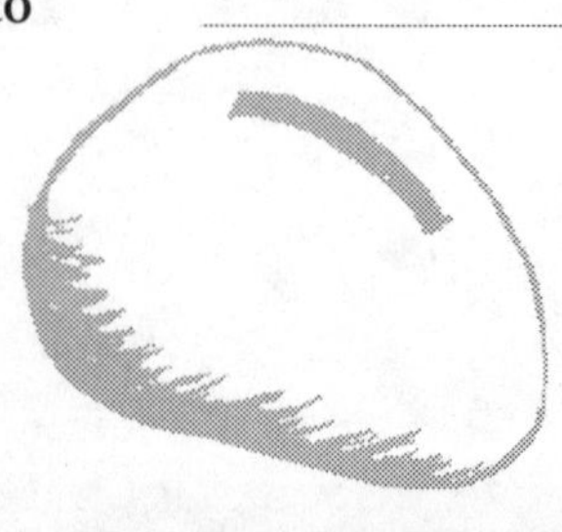

Apple Salsa

SERVES 2

2 firm Granny Smith apples
2 tbsp lemon juice
1 small chilli, seeded and finely chopped
1 tbsp oil
¼ cup raisins

CONVENTIONAL (5 MINUTES, PLUS STANDING TIME)

chopping board
knife
tablespoon
cup measure
apple corer
mixing bowl
spoon

1 PEEL, core and cut the apples into small dice, and place in a mixing bowl.
2 SQUEEZE the lemon juice over the apples, add the chilli, oil and raisins, and stir gently to mix evenly.
3 ALLOW to stand at room temperature for 30 minutes, if possible, to allow the flavours to develop.

Serve with pork, chicken, or burgers.

Mexican Salsa

SERVES 2

400 g firm ripe tomatoes
1 firm, ripe avocado
1 tbsp finely chopped white salad onion
1 tbsp chopped fresh coriander (or ¼ tsp dried)
2 tbsp lemon juice
dash of tabasco sauce

CONVENTIONAL (5 MINUTES, PLUS STANDING TIME)

chopping board
knife
tablespoon
lemon juicer
mixing bowl
spoon

1 HALVE the tomatoes and avocado, and remove the seeds and stone. Cut into small dice, and place in the mixing bowl.
2 ADD the onion, coriander and lemon juice, and stir through.
3 ALLOW to stand at room temperature for 30 minutes, if possible, to allow the flavours to develop.

Serve with fish, chicken, or oysters in the shell.

HG's Custard Caper

SERVES 2

2 tbsp custard powder
1 tbsp sugar
1½ cups low-fat milk
1 tsp vanilla essence (optional)

CONVENTIONAL (7 MINUTES)

tablespoon
cup measure
teaspoon
saucepan
wooden spoon

1 MAKE the custard according to the directions on the packet.

Serve sprinkled with chopped nuts or grated chocolate.

MICROWAVE (7 MINUTES)

tablespoon
cup measure
teaspoon
small microwave-safe container
spoon

1 MIX the custard powder and sugar with a little milk in the microwave-safe container until smooth and lump free. Add the remaining milk and vanilla.
2 COOK, uncovered, on HIGH (100%) for 2 minutes. Stir. Cook for another 2 minutes, stirring every 30 seconds.
3 ALLOW to stand for 1 minute.

Serve sprinkled with chopped nuts or grated chocolate.

HANDY MAN HINT

To turn this custard into an egg custard, whisk an egg in at the end of cooking time. It will cook in the heat of the custard as it stands, without scrambling.

Lemon Curd Indulgence — Blokes Behaving Badly

SERVES 2

250 g butter, chopped
juice and grated rind of 3 lemons
½ cup sugar
2 (61 g) eggs, at room temperature
1 (125g) can passionfruit pulp

MICROWAVE (12 MINUTES)

1 PLACE the butter in a microwave-safe container. Cook, uncovered, on MEDIUM (50%) for 1–2 minutes.
2 PLACE all the ingredients, except the butter, in the microwave-safe bowl. Whisk until the ingredients are well combined, then gradually add the melted butter, stirring the mixture continuously until smooth.
3 COOK, uncovered, on MEDIUM (50–60%) for 5–6 minutes, stirring three times during the cooking time, until the mixture has thickened. Stir in the passionfruit.

Serve drizzled over pancakes.

scales
knife
lemon juicer
grater
cup measure
can opener
spoon
medium-sized microwave-safe container
microwave-safe bowl
whisk or fork

HANDY MAN HINTS

- *Curd will refrigerate, and keep for four weeks.*
- *Spread small amounts of curd over multigrain bread.*
- *Before squeezing lemons, place them in a microwave oven and zap on HIGH (100%) for 10–15 seconds. You will be rewarded with twice as much juice. If you do not have a microwave oven, roll the lemon backwards and forwards on the bench with the palm of your hand to break down the fibres for a similar result.*

FIT TIP *Use this sauce sparingly as the ingredients are truly an indulgence for special occasions.*

'Wrong 'un' Chocolate Fudge Sauce

Makes 1½ cups

250 g dark or milk chocolate buds
½ cup cream
2 tbsp white sugar
½ tsp vanilla essence (optional)

scales
cup measure
tablespoon
teaspoon
medium-sized microwave-safe container
spoon

MICROWAVE (5 MINUTES)

1 COMBINE all the ingredients in the microwave-safe container and stir to combine evenly.
2 COOK, uncovered, on MEDIUM (50%) for 2–3 minutes until the chocolate has melted, stirring halfway through the cooking time. (Do not cover the chocolate while heating, as it will stiffen.)
3 STIR through the sauce with a spoon, and you will find it thickens up.

Serve over icecream, or make a sundae by sprinkling some nuts of your choice over the icecream and Chocolate Fudge Sauce (page 177).

HANDY MAN HINT

Store leftover sauce in the refrigerator. Bring back to pouring consistency by heating in a microwave oven in an uncovered microwave-safe bowl on MEDIUM (50%) for 1–2 minutes.

VARIATION

To make a chocolate milkshake, add 1–2 tbsp chocolate sauce to a glass of cold milk, whisk well, and serve with a scoop of icecream.

SOUL FOOD

'A husband always prefers his wife's mother-in-law to his own'

— Anonymous.

Through the mists of time, Mum-cooked meals have become legendary! These contemporary desserts are 'like Mum used to make', but lighter and easier.

FIT FODDER If you are one of those people who just has to finish a meal with dessert or it is not a meal, look for options that are not only quick and convenient but also nutritious.

Fruit is always a good idea, and in summer, when there is plenty of variety, a platter of fresh fruit with low-fat fromage frais or yoghurt is very satisfying — sweet, but low in fat.

If you like traditional desserts, try them with low-fat toppings, such as ricotta cream, yoghurt, fromage frais or low-fat custard for a great calcium boost. Remember, too, that your evening meal should not be the largest meal of the day — eat dessert after lunch instead, to avoid overeating at night.

Easy-as-apple Pie

Serves 2–3

1 sheet puff pastry, defrosted
1 (425 g) can apple pie fruit
½ cup rolled oats
2 tbsp white or brown sugar
2 tsp cinnamon

can opener
cup measure
tablespoon
teaspoon
2 metal baking trays
baking paper

CONVENTIONAL (25 MINUTES)

Preheat the oven to 200°C.

1 COVER two metal baking trays with baking paper, and place a sheet of pastry on each. Cut each sheet into four squares.
2 PLACE a heaped tablespoonful of the apple in the middle of the squares, and sprinkle with oats, sugar and cinnamon. Moisten the edges with water, and fold in the four sides to make a parcel or envelope.
3 BAKE for 15 minutes, until the pastry is golden brown and crisp.

Serve with custard, cream or icecream.

HANDY MAN HINT

Use leftover pastry sheets to make Short-pass Savoury Cheese Squares (page 133).

Chocolate Cake

Serves 2

1 chocolate cake mix
2 (61 g) eggs
¾ cup low-fat milk
1 tbsp Marsala (optional)

CONVENTIONAL (15 MINUTES)

mixing bowl
beaters
cup measure
tablespoon
cake pan
wire rack

1 COOK the cake according to the directions on the packet. Include the Marsala if desired.

Serve with custard (page 154) or coulis (page 166).

MICROWAVE (12 MINUTES)

mixing bowl
beaters or fork
cup measure
tablespoon
medium-sized microwave-safe container
non-recycled paper towel
microwave-safe saucer

1 PLACE the cake mix in a bowl, and add the eggs, Marsala (if desired) and milk. Mix the ingredients together with a fork for 2 minutes until evenly combined. Do not overbeat.
2 LINE the base of the microwave-safe container with paper towel. Pour in the cake mixture, and cover loosely with paper towel.
3 PLACE the container on an upturned saucer in the centre of the turntable, and cook on HIGH (100%) for 6 minutes. Allow to stand for 5 minutes.

Serve with custard (page 154) or coulis (page 166).

HANDY MAN HINT

Overbeating cakes to be cooked in the microwave results in a tough cake with large holes through it.

VARIATION

Turn this cake into a 'Bowled' Berry Pudding (page 160).

'Bowled' Berry Pudding

Serves 2

1 punnet of fresh strawberries, rinsed, hulled and cut into quarters
150 g fresh or frozen blueberries
2 tbsp castor sugar
¼ cup water
2 large slices Chocolate Cake (page 159)
2 scoops low-fat icecream

CONVENTIONAL (15 MINUTES)

colander
chopping board
knife
tablespoon
cup measure
small saucepan
icecream scoop

1 COMBINE the berries, sugar and water in the saucepan, and bring the mixture to the boil over medium heat. Simmer for 1 minute.
2 REMOVE from the heat, and place the saucepan in the fridge or freezer for 10 minutes to cool.
3 ASSEMBLE: place a cake slice in each bowl, and top with the berry mixture and a scoop of icecream.

MICROWAVE (15 MINUTES)

colander
chopping board
knife
tablespoon
cup measure
small microwave-safe container
icecream scoop

1 COMBINE the berries, sugar and water in the microwave-safe container. Cover, and cook on HIGH (100%) for 2 minutes.
2 ALLOW to stand for several minutes, then place the container in the fridge or freezer to cool for 10 minutes.
3 ASSEMBLE: place a cake slice in each bowl, and top with the berry mixture and a scoop of icecream.

HANDY MAN HINTS

- *Fresh blueberries are available during summer. Add them to cereal as an energy booster for breakfast.*
- *Soften frozen icecream in a microwave oven on HIGH (100%) for 30 seconds to make it easy to scoop and serve.*

Baked Apples with Attitude

Serves 2

4 Granny Smith apples, cored
2 tbsp honey
2 tbsp natural muesli
1 orange: rind grated, then juiced

CONVENTIONAL (50 MINUTES)

chopping board
apple corer
tablespoon
grater
lemon juicer
fork or skewer
baking dish
mixing bowl
spoon

Preheat the oven to 180°C.

1 PIERCE the skins of the apples several times with a fork or skewer, and place the apples in the baking dish.
2 MIX the honey, muesli, grated rind of the orange and the juice in the bowl. Fill the cavity of each apple with the mixture.
3 BAKE the apples for 45 minutes until they are soft but the skin has not split.

Serve with custard (page 154).

MICROWAVE (10 MINUTES)

chopping board
apple corer
tablespoon
grater
lemon juicer
fork or skewer
medium-sized microwave-safe container
mixing bowl
spoon
non-recycled paper towel

1 PIERCE the skins of the apples several times with a fork or skewer, and place the apples around the edge of the microwave-safe container.
2 MIX the honey, muesli, grated rind of the orange and the juice in a bowl. Fill the cavity of each apple with the mixture.
3 COVER with paper towel, and cook on HIGH (100%) for 5–6 minutes. Pour the juice back over the apples, and allow to stand for 1 minute.

Serve with custard (page 154).

HANDY MAN HINT *Stew apples in their skins to retain more flavour and vitamins. Pierce the apple skin several times with a fork or skewer, place in the microwave oven, and cook, uncovered, on HIGH (100%) for 3 minutes. Scoop out the pulp and serve this over cereal or icecream.*

VARIATION *Try other fillings such as dried fruit, or diced apricot with pine nuts.*

Perfect Pancakes

SERVES 2

1 cup plain flour
1 cup low-fat milk
1 (55 g) egg
pinch of salt (optional)
1 tsp oil
2 large lemons, cut into quarters
2 tbsp sugar

CONVENTIONAL (1½ HOURS)

cup measure
tablespoon
medium-sized jug
fork
non-stick frypan
egg lifter
warmed plate

1 COMBINE the first four ingredients in a jug, and mix with a fork until the mixture is smooth. Allow the batter to stand for at least 1 hour before using, longer if possible.
2 LIGHTLY oil a preheated frypan, and put over medium heat. Spoon 2 heaped tbsp batter mixture into the centre of the frypan, tilting the pan to allow mixture to spread. Cook the pancake for 1–2 minutes until the surface bubbles, and edges lift.
3 PLACE the cooked pancake on a warmed plate.
Repeat the procedure until all the batter is used.
Serve with a squeeze of lemon juice, and a sprinkling of sugar.

HANDY MAN HINTS

- *Pancakes freeze successfully.*
- *Serve sweet with golden syrup, maple syrup or fruit spread, or savoury spread with light sour cream, smoked salmon and dill pickles.*

Fast-track Banana Custard

SERVES 2

2 tbsp custard powder
1 tbsp sugar
1½ cups low-fat milk
1 tsp vanilla essence (optional)
1 banana, peeled and sliced

CONVENTIONAL (7 MINUTES)

1 MAKE the custard according to the directions on the packet.
2 ADD the sliced banana to the custard.

Serve sprinkled with cinnamon or crushed nuts.

tablespoon
cup measure
teaspoon
chopping board
knife
saucepan
wooden spoon

MICROWAVE (5 MINUTES)

1 MIX the custard powder and sugar with a little milk in the microwave-safe container until smooth and lump free. Add the remaining milk and vanilla.
2 COOK, uncovered, on HIGH (100%) for 2 minutes. Stir. Cook for another 2 minutes, stirring every 30 seconds.
3 ADD the sliced banana to the custard. Allow to stand for 1 minute.

Serve sprinkled with cinnamon or crushed nuts.

tablespoon
cup measure
teaspoon
chopping board
knife
small microwave-safe container
spoon

HANDY MAN HINT

To turn this custard into an egg custard, whisk in an egg at the end of the cooking time. It will cook in the heat of the custard, as it stands, without scrambling.

'Stoned' Dried Fruit Salad

SERVES 2

300 g mixed dried fruit of your choice (apricots, apples, sultanas, mixed fruit, raisins, peaches, etc.)
1 cup apple juice
2 tbsp sugar
½ cup sweet white wine (or water)
1 tsp vanilla

CONVENTIONAL (20 MINUTES)

scales
cup measure
tablespoon
teaspoon
wide-based saucepan
wooden spoon

1 COMBINE all the ingredients in the saucepan, and stir over medium heat for 6–8 minutes until the sugar is dissolved.
2 SIMMER over medium heat for a further 8–10 minutes, stirring once.

Serve warm or cold with low-fat yoghurt or icecream.

MICROWAVE (12 MINUTES)

scales
cup measure
tablespoon
teaspoon
medium-sized microwave-safe container, and lid
spoon

1 COMBINE all the ingredients in the microwave-safe container. Cover, and cook on HIGH (100%) for 4 minutes.
2 STIR. Cover, and cook on HIGH (100%) for a further 4 minutes. Allow to stand for 2 minutes.

Serve warm or cold with low-fat icecream or yoghurt.

HANDY MAN HINT

Keep leftover fruit salad in the fridge, and use over cereal or yoghurt for a great power breakfast.

Icecream Sundae Event

SERVES 2

500 ml low-fat vanilla icecream
1 cup Strawberry Coulis (page 166)
½ cup thickened cream or fromage frais
2 tbsp crushed nuts (walnuts or pecans)

cup measure
tablespoon
icecream scoop (or spoon)
2 long glasses

CONVENTIONAL (10 MINUTES)

1 PLACE scoops of icecream in large glasses.
2 POUR the strawberry coulis over.
3 TOP with cream, and sprinkle with nuts.

VARIATIONS

- *Add some fresh fruit to the topping, e.g. sliced bananas, mango or kiwi fruit.*
- *Add some crushed choc-mint bars or 'hundreds 'n' thousands' for some perennial favourites among the kids in your family.*
- *Place seasonal fresh berrries or fruit in a container, and pour slightly cooled jelly mix over. Leave to set in a fridge, and serve a scoop of jellied fruit with a scoop of low-fat icecream for a refreshing dessert.*

Sinking Shots with Strawberry Coulis

Serves 2

1 (420 g) can strawberries or raspberries, drained (or 400 g frozen)
1 tbsp sugar
juice of ½ lemon
1 tbsp sherry or Grand Marnier (optional)
2 tbsp crushed nuts

CONVENTIONAL (5 MINUTES)

can opener
strainer
tablespoon
lemon juicer
blender (or fork and mixing bowl)
icecream scoop (or spoon)

1 PLACE all the ingredients in a blender, and process until well combined.

Serve over the icecream of your choice, and sprinkle with crushed nuts.

MICROWAVE (4 MINUTES)

can opener
strainer
tablespoon
lemon juicer
small microwave-safe bowl
fork
icecream scoop (or spoon)

1 COMBINE all the ingredients in the microwave-safe bowl. Cook, uncovered, on HIGH (100%) for 2 minutes to soften.
2 MASH the mixture with a fork until it is smooth.

Serve over the icecream of your choice, and sprinkle with crushed nuts.

HANDY MAN HINTS

- *Fresh strawberries are low in fat, and are a good source of vitamin C.*
- *Do not wash strawberries until you are ready to use them.*
- *Strawberries freeze very well, and make a good iced snack on a hot day.*
- *If fresh berries are not in season, use frozen berries.*

VARIATION *Use other canned berries instead of strawberries or raspberries.*

Masters' Cheesecake

SERVES 8

2 (250 g) blocks light cream cheese
½ cup castor sugar
½ cup cream
3 tsp gelatine, dissolved in ¼ cup boiling water
½ cup chopped nuts

CONVENTIONAL (1 HOUR 40 MINUTES)

cup measure
teaspoon
chopping board
knife
beaters or fork
mixing bowl
small jug or cup
spoon
medium-sized container or cake tin

1 BEAT the cheese until it is smooth. Add the sugar, cream and dissolved gelatine mixture, and beat well until evenly combined.
2 POUR the mixture into the container, and sprinkle with the nuts.
3 REFRIGERATE for 1½ hours until the mixture sets.

Serve slices with fruit, such as grapes, strawberries or raisins.

HANDY MAN HINT *Soften cream cheese in a microwave oven on HIGH (100%) for 45 seconds, to make it easier to beat.*

FIT TIP *Measure your waist size every week, and keep a record of it. Focus on your behaviour rather than on your weight — how you eat and exercise, rather than what you weigh.*

VARIATION *For a chocolate cheesecake, drizzle 2 tbsp chocolate topping over the cheesecake before putting it in the fridge.*

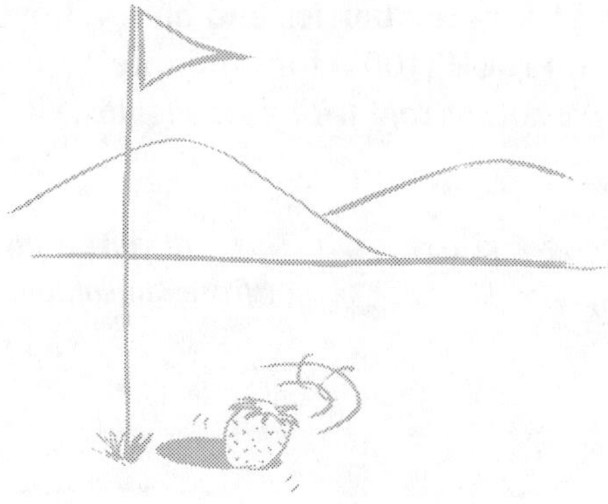

Flash Fruit Salad

Serves 2

2 large ripe peaches
2 large nectarines
2 plums
2 cups water (conventional method);
 1 cup water (microwave)
2 tbsp honey
1 punnet strawberries
low-fat fruit yoghurt

CONVENTIONAL (20 MINUTES)

knife
chopping board
cup measure
large saucepan
wooden spoon
tablespoon

1 LEAVING the fruit unpeeled, cut around and discard the stone, then chop the peaches into six, the nectarines into four, and the plums in half.
2 ADD the fruit and water to the saucepan, and bring to the boil over high heat. Then simmer over low heat for 15 minutes.
3 STIR in the berries and honey, and cook for a further minute.

Serve hot, or cold with fruit yoghurt.

MICROWAVE (10 MINUTES)

knife
chopping board
cup measure
large microwave-
 safe container,
 and lid
spoon
tablespoon

1 LEAVING the fruit unpeeled, cut around and discard the stone, then chop the peaches into six, the nectarines into four, and the plums in half.
2 PLACE the prepared fruit in the microwave-safe container, and pour in the water. Cover, and cook on HIGH (100%) for 5 minutes.
3 STIR in the berries and honey. Cover, and cook on HIGH (100%) for 1 minute.

Serve hot, or cold with fruit yoghurt.

HANDY MAN HINT

This fruit can be stored for one week in the refrigerator, or frozen in containers to extend the season.

Married to the Mob

'Parents are sometimes a disappointment to their children. They don't fulfil the promise of their early years'

— Anthony Powell.

Irrespective of your status, somewhere along the line you are likely to be confronted by kids in a kitchen, yours, hers, theirs, etc. These are quick and easy recipes for future kitchen aerobics.

Fit Tips Cooking nutritious food for kids is incredibly simple. With a little imagination you can have children 'eating out of your hands', and taking the pressure off you for trips to Macca's or KFC every weekend.

Important nutrients for growing children include protein and calcium, which are found in abundant quantities in dairy foods. Encourage your children to eat cheese, milk and yoghurt regularly by offering it in a variety of ways — cheese on toast, milk smoothies, yoghurt, fruit, etc.

Kids' Grub

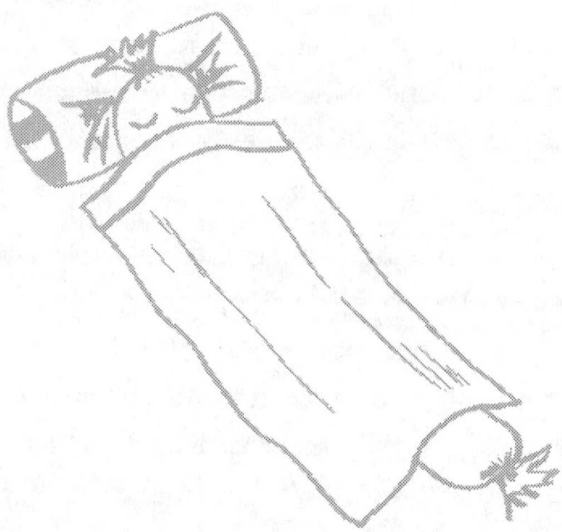

Pizza Muffins

Serves 2

4 English muffins, halved
4 tbsp mild taco sauce
4 slices lean ham, finely chopped
4 tbsp grated mozzarella cheese

CONVENTIONAL (6 MINUTES)

chopping board
knife
tablespoon
grater

1 TOAST the muffin halves on both sides.
2 SPREAD the muffins with taco sauce. Sprinkle with ham on top, then the cheese. Place the prepared muffins under a preheated hot grill, and cook for 2–3 minutes until the cheese is golden brown.

MICROWAVE (8 MINUTES)

chopping board
knife
tablespoon
grater
non-recycled paper towel
microwave-safe dinner plate

1 SPREAD the muffin halves with taco sauce. Sprinkle the ham on top, and then the cheese.
2 PLACE a sheet of paper towel on a dinner plate, and arrange the muffins on top. Cook, uncovered, on HIGH (100%) for 1–1½ minutes per muffin, or 4 minutes for 4 muffins.

HANDY MAN HINT

Toast a pack of muffins, and keep frozen ready to thaw for snacks. Kids love them spread with vegemite, or strawberry jam.

Egg 'n' Bacon Noodles

SERVES 2–4

4–5 cups water
1 (250 g) pkt Chinese noodles
2 middle rashers lean rindless bacon, chopped
2 (55 g) eggs
½ cup grated tasty cheese

chopping board
knife
grater
large saucepan
  and lid
colander
non-stick frypan
wooden spoon
paper towel
egg lifter
serving spoon

CONVENTIONAL (12 MINUTES)

1 PLACE the water in the saucepan and bring to the boil. Add the noodles, and cook according to the directions on the packet. Drain the noodles, and cover to keep them warm.
2 HEAT the frypan over medium heat, add the bacon, and cook over medium heat for 2 minutes, stirring occasionally. Drain the bacon on paper towel.
3 BREAK the eggs into the warm pan, and cook over medium heat for 3–4 minutes until the yolks are hard. Slice the cooked eggs, then toss them through the noodles with the bacon.

Serve the noodle mixture in bowls, top with the cheese, and with cherry tomatoes as a salad.

VARIATION *Use finely-sliced lean ham instead of bacon.*

Baked Bean-bag

1 (225 g) can low-salt baked beans
2 tbsp frozen peas
1 tbsp grated tasty cheese

SERVES 1

CONVENTIONAL (5 MINUTES)

1 PLACE the beans and peas in a small saucepan. Warm over a low heat for 2 to 3 minutes, stirring halfway through the cooking time.
2 SPRINKLE the cheese over the top, and allow to stand for 1 minute to melt the cheese.

Allow to cool slightly before serving.

can opener
tablespoon
grater
small saucepan
wooden spoon

MICROWAVE (3 MINUTES)

1 PLACE the beans and peas in the microwave-safe container. Cook, uncovered, on HIGH (100%) for 1½ minutes.
2 SPRINKLE the cheese over the top, and cook on HIGH (100%) for 30 seconds to melt the cheese.

Allow to cool slightly before serving.

can opener
tablespoon
grater
small microwave safe container

Pig in Bed

SERVES 1

1 low-fat sausage, cooked
1 slice high-fibre bread
1 tbsp tomato sauce
1 tbsp grated cheese

CONVENTIONAL (4 MINUTES)

1 WRAP the cooked sausage in the bread, and add the sauce on top.
2 SPRINKLE with the cheese, and place under a preheated grill for 1–2 minutes, until the cheese melts.

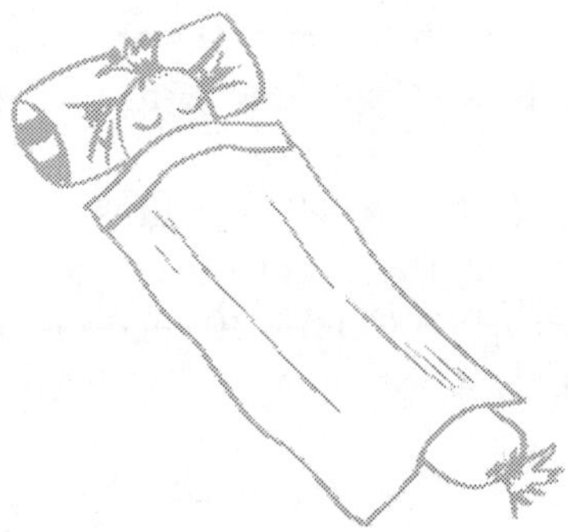

Spaghetti Face

SERVES 1

1 (225 g) can spaghetti
3 cherry tomatoes
1 carrot stick, cut into small strips
1 stick celery, cut into small strips
1 mushroom, sliced

CONVENTIONAL (5 MINUTES)

1 PLACE the ingredients on a dinner plate to create a face: face (spaghetti), hair (carrot and celery sticks), eyes and nose (cherry tomatoes), mouth (mushroom slices).

Serve with a smile!

can opener
spoon
chopping board
knife
potato peeler

Ankle Biters' Cocktail Snack Attack

SERVES 3–6

1 (500 g) pkt cocktail frankfurts, each pierced several times with a fork
water (conventional method only)

CONVENTIONAL (10 MINUTES)

fork
saucepan
knife or scissors
colander
serving tongs

1 FOLLOW the directions given on the packet.

Serve with tomato sauce.

MICROWAVE (5 MINUTES)

knife or scissors
serving tongs

1 PLACE the prepared frankfurts around the edge of the turntable, making two circles, one inside the other.
2 COOK on HIGH (100%) for 3 minutes. Allow to stand for 1 minute.

Serve with tomato sauce.

VARIATION *Serve on cocktail skewers topped with pineapple pieces.*

Time-out Chocolate Fudge Crackle

½ cup Chocolate Fudge Sauce (page 177)
2 cups Rice Bubbles

MAKES 8

MICROWAVE (5 MINUTES)

1 COMBINE the sauce and rice bubbles in the microwave-safe container.
2 MIX the ingredients until evenly combined, then smooth the mixture flat in the container.
3 REFRIGERATE until set, and then cut into squares.

cup measure
large microwave-safe container
spoon
knife

HANDY MAN HINT *Always store chocolate covered, as it very quickly absorbs other odours, such as onion.*

VARIATION *Add chopped nuts or dried fruit.*

Chocolate Fudge Sauce

MAKES 1½ CUPS

250 g dark or milk chocolate buds
½ cup cream
2 tbsp white sugar
½ tsp vanilla essence (optional)

- scales
- cup measure
- tablespoon
- teaspoon
- medium-sized microwave-safe glass container
- icecream scoop or spoon

MICROWAVE (6 MINUTES)

1 COMBINE all the ingredients in the microwave-safe glass container, and stir to combine evenly.
2 COOK on MEDIUM (50%) for 2–3 minutes until the chocolate has melted, stirring halfway through the cooking time. (Do not cover the chocolate during cooking, as it will stiffen.)
3 STIR through the sauce to thicken it up.

Serve over icecream.

VARIATION *Turn this into a sundae by sprinkling some nuts of your choice over the icecream and sauce.*

Strawberry Snacks

Nothing tastes as good as a luscious, freshly-picked strawberry — and to think this indulgence is actually good for your kids!

Choose fully-coloured strawberries that are firm, bright and plump. Store them in the fridge in a bowl lined with absorbent paper. Wash the strawberries just before use (this prevents water breaking down the flavour and texture), and remove (huli) the green tops.

Here's the healthy part: strawberries are an excellent source of vitamin C and are low in fat and kilojoules — even more reason for your 'mob' to discover the joys of snacking on strawberries any time, every day. Fresh strawberries also freeze very well for out-of-season snacks.

Playing Games

'What's life about? Life is about filling in the time with different things before you die'

— Sam Newman.

Whether you are a player or a playboy or just a spectator, you need to know what to eat and drink after playing sport or spending a day in the sun as an onlooker.

High-performance tips The right diet is critical for optimal performance on the sporting field. Muscles need enough carbohydrate in storage (known as glycogen) to sustain regular exercise, and this comes from your diet. Eat more rice, pasta, bread, potatoes, fruit, legumes and breakfast cereals, as inadequate carbohydrate will leave you feeling tired during exercise, and will prevent proper recovery after strenuous exercise.

Base all your meals and snacks on high-carbohydrate foods. A high-fat diet will contribute to high body-fat levels and will prevent you eating enough carbohydrate. Avoid added fats such as butter and margarine, cook without added oils, avoid fried foods, and choose low-fat dairy foods and lean meat and poultry. Eat carbo-snacks immediately after recovery from training or competition, and drink plenty of fluid over the day — at least 2 litres of water, with a little cordial, fruit juice and sports drinks for variety.

Perfect Pre-gamers

Sports Smoothies (page 181)
Club Sandwich (page 182)
The Ace of Spuds (page 56)
Perfect Pancakes (page 162)

Most people find it difficult to eat a lot before exercising, particularly where the activity involves rapid movements of the body, as in running, racquet sports, football, etc. Drinks such as smoothies, and plain sandwiches, make good pre-game meals. For those who are a little hungrier, baked beans provide a sustained source of carbohydrate — however, practise eating them before training first, to make sure the wind-power factor is not too strong!

Winter Warm-down

Pasta 'n' Pumpkin Soup (page 183)
Hommus Skinny Dip (page 184)
Some-like-it-hot Mexican Rice (page 48)

Pumpkin, like potato, is a vegetable rich in carbohydrates and also a great source of the antioxidant vitamin A. Add some pasta and toast, and you have a super high-carbohydrate meal that takes minutes to prepare, and is perfect for recovery after a cold winter's night's training.

Spectator Snacks

Game, Set and Match (page 185)
Crumpet Pizza League (page 186)

When your event has finished and you're watching everyone else, instead of foraging through the fast-food outlets at the venue, bring your own high-performance foods to save money and your health.

Carbo Loading

Tomato Pasta Authentico (page 187)
Crusty roll
Sam's Passion Punch (page 188)

For endurance exercise lasting more than 1½ hours (e.g. marathon, triathlon, skiing), it is useful to 'superload' the muscles' glycogen stores by having a very high carbohydrate intake for three days before your competition. A sports dietitian can plan a personalised carbohydrate-loading programme for you, to ensure you meet your energy needs.

Sports Smoothies

CONVENTIONAL (5 MINUTES)

SERVES 1

Place all the ingredients in a blender, and blend until smooth.

Banana Smoothie

250 ml cold low-fat milk
1 banana, chopped
pulp of 1 passionfruit
1 tsp honey

cup measure
chopping board
knife
teaspoon
blender, or fork and mixing bowl

Nutty Banana Whiz

250 ml cold low-fat milk
1 banana, chopped
1 tsp peanut butter
2 tsp honey

cup measure
chopping board
knife
teaspoon
blender, or fork and mixing bowl

Strawberry Crush

250 ml cold low-fat milk
½ cup strawberries, washed and hulled
1 (250 g) tub low-fat berry yoghurt
1 tsp honey

cup measure
knife
spoon
teaspoon
blender, or fork and mixing bowl

Iced Coffee

250 ml cold low-fat milk
1 tsp instant coffee
1 tbsp honey

cup measure
teaspoon
tablespoon
blender, or fork and mixing bowl

Troppo Super Shake

250 ml cold low-fat milk
½ cup crushed pineapple, well drained
1 (250 g) tub light tropical fruit yoghurt
2 tsp honey

cup measure
can opener
strainer
spoon
teaspoon
blender, or fork and mixing bowl

HANDY MAN HINT *For the best results, make sure all the ingredients are icy cold.*

VARIATION *Add 1 (250 g) tub of low-fat yoghurt to those recipes without yoghurt already.*

Club Sandwich — for the Men in White

SERVES 2

4 slices wholemeal bread
2 slices multigrain bread
4 tbsp jam (e.g. strawberry, plum or fig)
4 tbsp ricotta cheese

CONVENTIONAL

tablespoon
knife

1 SPREAD two slices of wholemeal bread with jam, and cover with the multigrain bread.
2 SPREAD the top slices with the cheese, and cover with remaining wholemeal bread.

Cut the sandwich in half to serve.

HANDY MAN HINTS

- *Store a sliced loaf of bread in a plastic bag in the freezer.*
- *Take out only as many slices as you need, and reseal the bag.*
- *To defrost sliced bread quickly: place two slices of bread on a sheet of non-recycled paper towel, and defrost on HIGH (100%) for 15–20 seconds.*

VARIATION *Vary your bread; there are now many delicious varieties of grain bread at local bakeries.*

Pasta 'n' Pumpkin Soup

SERVES 2

1 small butternut pumpkin (500 g), peeled and cubed (conventional method); left whole (microwave)
2 cups vegetable stock, hot
2 spring onions, finely chopped
1 cup cooked pasta
2 tsp nutmeg
½ cup low-fat milk, at room temperature

CONVENTIONAL (30 MINUTES)

chopping board
knife
cup measure
teaspoon
large saucepan
blender or fork
wooden spoon
soup ladle

1 PLACE the pumpkin and stock in the saucepan, cover and bring to the boil. Simmer over medium heat for 15 minutes or until the pumpkin is soft.
2 COOL the soup, and place it in a blender or whisk with a fork. Blend for 1–2 minutes, before returning to the saucepan with the onions, pasta and nutmeg.
3 STIR in the milk and pasta, and reheat over medium heat for 3 minutes until warm, but do not boil.

Serve with crusty bread.

MICROWAVE (25 MINUTES)

chopping board
knife
cup measure
teaspoon
fork
microwave-safe dinner plate
spoon
large microwave-safe container, and lid
soup ladle

1 PIERCE the pumpkin six times with a fork, and place on an upturned microwave-safe dinner plate. Cook on HIGH (100%) for 10–12 minutes until the flesh is soft. Test with a skewer. Allow to stand for 5 minutes to cool.
2 CUT the pumpkin in half lengthwise, and scoop the flesh into the microwave-safe container. Add the stock, onions, pasta and nutmeg.
3 COVER, and cook on HIGH (100%) for 4 minutes, stirring halfway through the cooking time. Stir in the milk.

Serve with crusty bread.

VARIATIONS

- *Add curry instead of nutmeg.*
- *Add ½ cup sweetcorn kernels or canned prawns or 1 tbsp of mixed fresh herbs, chopped.*
- *Replace the milk or cream with 1 tbsp natural yoghurt.*

Hommus Skinny Dip

Serves 2

1 (440 g) can chick peas, well drained
2 cloves garlic, peeled and crushed
⅓ cup lemon juice
2 tsp soy sauce

can opener
strainer
spoon
chopping board
knife
cup measure
lemon juicer
teaspoon
blender or fork

CONVENTIONAL (5 MINUTES)

1 COMBINE all the ingredients in a blender, or whisk in a bowl with a fork, until smooth.

Serve on toast or brown bread. Delicious as a dip with Pita Chips (page 136) or fingers of celery and carrots.

HANDY MAN HINT

Remember that dried beans need some forward planning before eating them (see pages 109–10), although most beans are now available in cans from supermarkets.

VARIATIONS

- *Hommus is delicious as a spread for sandwiches.*
- *Add ½ cup tahini to the ingredients.*

Game, Set and Match

2 tbsp peanut butter
1 tbsp raisins
2 wholemeal muffins, split in half

SERVES 2

CONVENTIONAL (5 MINUTES)

1 MASH the peanut butter and raisins together in a mixing bowl with a fork.
2 TOAST the muffins.
3 SPREAD the muffin halves with the peanut mixture.

tablespoon
mixing bowl
fork
toaster
plate
table knife

HANDY MAN HINT

Bananas freeze well. They make a terrific alternative to an icecream snack if first rolled in fruit juice, and then in crushed nuts. Freezing takes approximately 4 hours.

VARIATIONS

- *Omit the raisins, and mash a banana together with the peanut butter.*
- *Spread the toasted muffins with Hommus Skinny Dip (page 184).*

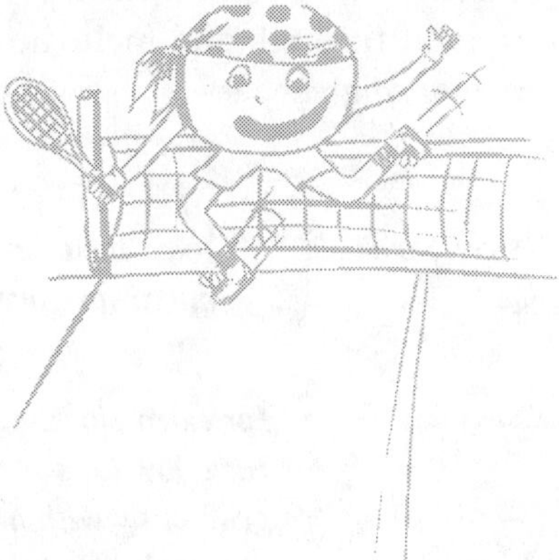

Crumpet Pizza League

SERVES 2

2 tsp margarine (conventional method only)
4 crumpets
4 tbsp your favourite pasta sauce
4 tbsp low-fat grated tasty cheese
2 tbsp chopped olives

CONVENTIONAL (10 MINUTES)

1 MELT the margarine in the frypan over low heat. Place the crumpets in the pan, and spread with pasta sauce, sprinkle with the cheese, and top with olives.
2 COOK over low heat for 5–6 minutes, until the crumpets are warmed through and the cheese has melted.

Serve immediately.

teaspoon
tablespoon
grater
chopping board
knife
non-stick frypan

MICROWAVE (6 MINUTES)

1 PLACE the crumpets in the microwave-safe container. Spread with the pasta sauce, sprinkle with the cheese and top with the olives.
2 COVER, and cook on HIGH (100%) for 3 minutes to heat through and melt the cheese.

Serve immediately.

teaspoon
tablespoon
grater
chopping board
knife
large microwave safe container, and lid

HANDY MAN HINT

Toast the crumpets first for a crisper finish in a microwave oven.

VARIATIONS

- *For extra zip, use taco sauce instead of pasta sauce.*
- *For a low-fat sweet treat, toast the crumpets and spread generously with honey and top with sliced banana. Leave out the butter to make this a no-fat snack.*

Tomato Pasta Authentico

SERVES 2

560 g pasta, cooked

Sauce

1 onion, roughly chopped
1 clove garlic, crushed
1 tsp dried basil
1 tbsp oil
1 (425 g) can Italian-style tomatoes
2 tsp sugar

CONVENTIONAL (25 MINUTES)

large saucepan, and lid
colander
chopping board
knife
teaspoon
tablespoon
can opener
wooden spoon

1 BRING a large saucepan of water to the boil, add the pasta, and cook according to the directions on the packet. Drain, cover and keep pasta warm.
2 COMBINE the onion, garlic, basil and oil in the saucepan, and cook over medium heat for 5–6 minutes. Add the tomatoes and sugar, and roughly chop through with a knife. Cook over medium heat, uncovered, for 5 minutes. Stir once halfway through the cooking time.
3 STIR in the cooked hot pasta, mixing together evenly.

Serve with a crusty roll.

MICROWAVE (25 MINUTES)

large saucepan, and lid
colander
chopping board
knife
teaspoon
tablespoon
can opener
large microwave-safe container
spoon

1 BRING a large saucepan of water to the bowl, add the pasta and cook according to the directions on the packet. Drain, and keep the pasta warm.
2 COMBINE the onion, garlic, basil and oil in the microwave-safe container, and cook, uncovered, on HIGH (100%) for 4 minutes.
3 ADD the tomatoes and sugar, and roughly chop through with a knife. Cook, uncovered, on HIGH (100%) for 2–3 minutes.
4 STIR in the cooked hot pasta, mixing together evenly.

Serve with a crusty roll.

Sam's Passion Punch

SERVES 1

2 slices fresh or canned pineapple
2 oranges, peeled and chopped
dash water
pulp of 1 passionfruit

CONVENTIONAL (5 MINUTES)

1 COMBINE all the ingredients in a blender.
2 BLEND until smooth.

Serve in a chilled long glass. Here's luck!

can opener (if using canned pineapple)
chopping board
knife
teaspoon
blender
long glass

HANDY MAN HINT

To make oranges easier to peel, place them in a microwave oven, and cook on HIGH (100%) for 25 seconds.

VARIATION

Use easy-to-peel tangelos in place of the oranges.

THE 'F' WORD

'Peel me a grape, Beulah'

— Mae West.

Surveys have shown that many men do not eat fruit unless it is peeled for them. Here are some suggestions on how to use popular fruits without peeling or working overtime, and to add essential fibre, vitamins and minerals to your day. Dried fruit are delicious too, though you have to open a packet!

FIT TIPS

Fruit is rich in vitamins A and C, both potent antioxidants. Antioxidants prevent oxidative damage in your body, caused by factors such as pollution, environmental stresses and strenuous exercise. All men should aim to eat at least three pieces of fruit a day; if you exercise regularly, increase that to four or five pieces, minimum.

Fruit is very high in the carbohydrate fructose, has loads of dietary fibre, and most fruit has no fat at all!

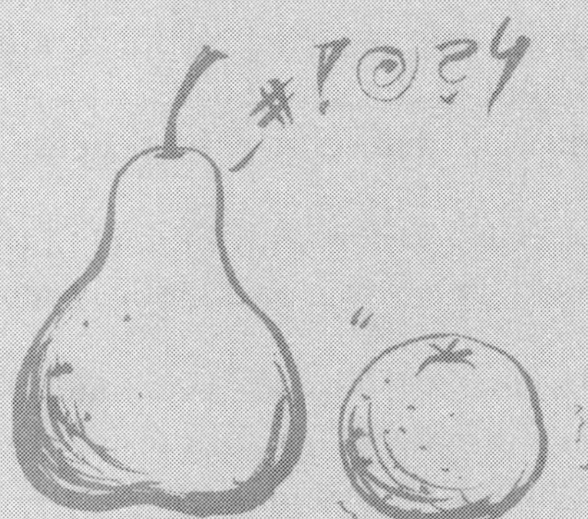

Apples: They are the best convenience food, and you have eighty varieties to choose from! Eat them straight, bake them (page 161), chop them into a fruit salad or fruit 'n' nut mixture (page 194), or turn them into a salsa (page 153) with lemon juice, finely chopped chilli and a drizzle of light olive oil.

Apricots: A sure sign of summer, apricots are small and succulent, and a snack-sized treat. Poach them with cinnamon in water or wine, and serve with icecream or yoghurt. Good when cold over cereal too.

Grapes: If you have no one to peel them for you, freeze them for summer iced 'bytes'. Dip them in egg white and roll them in castor sugar to frost them for a special fruit platter.

Melon trifecta: Melons are best cut into wedges. Watermelons are low in kilojoules, and a great thirst quencher. Honeydew melons are available all year round, so snack on them any time. Canteloupes (or rock melons), are delicious on their own, or remove the seeds and serve with finely sliced prosciutto. Mix pieces or balls of the three melons together for a summer cooler.

Oranges: You can make your own fresh juice instantly. Oranges freeze well too: cut them into wedges and freeze for a pick-me-up to eat any time.

Peaches: A luscious fruit, peaches are wonderful as a finish to a meal. To make an instant 'peach melba', halve the fruit, remove the stone, fill each half with icecream, and top with strawberry puree (page 166).

Pears: They are the ideal food for busy or stressed people, as they provide energy-giving carbohydrate and fluid, and are great after a workout in the gym. Slice, add a squeeze of lemon juice to prevent browning, and serve with a cheese platter.

Pineapples: Laden with vitamin C, they are now available, ready peeled, in cryovac packs. Slice them, and throw them on the barbie!

Strawberries: These are everyone's favourite snack food, and delicious sliced or halved in drinks too. They are cheap in summer, so take advantage of this: fold 1 punnet of strawberries (washed, hulled and sliced) into 1 litre softened low-fat vanilla icecream, and refreeze to serve in cones as a summer cooler.

Tangelos: These are a cross between a mandarine and a grapefruit, and are very easy to peel. They are distinguished from other citrus fruits by their deep orange colour. Add finely grated tangelo rind to mashed potato — sensational!

HANDY MAN HINT

Soften icecream on HIGH (100%) for 30 seconds in the microwave oven to make it easy to scoop or to mix with fruit before refreezing.

Blueberry and Mango Tango

SERVES 2

1 mango, peeled and sliced
1 punnet fresh or frozen blueberries
1 tbsp low-fat yoghurt

CONVENTIONAL (5 MINUTES)

chopping board
potato peeler
knife
2 bowls
tablespoon

1 PLACE slices of fresh mango in each bowl, and top with fresh or frozen blueberries.
2 ADD a swirl of yoghurt to each.

Serve immediately.

HANDY MAN HINTS

The mango has a large flat stone, and so must be cut in a certain way. Follow these four simple steps:

- *Peel the mango with a potato peeler or, if the mango is sufficiently ripe, pull the skin down from the stem end (like peeling a banana). Place the mango on a chopping board, and cut slices from both flatter sides of the fruit, as close to the stone as possible.*
- *Slice any other flesh from around the stone.*
- *Cut the flesh into slices (or cubes).*

VARIATION

Mangoes are most people's favourite fruit, and are versatile enough to mix with many other summer and winter fruits.

FIT TIP

For the weight conscious it is reassuring to know that a 100 g serve of mango provides just 268 Kj — so you can go ahead and indulge at the end of the meal!

Fruit and Nuts

SERVES 2

small pkts dried fruit
nashi pears
nuts (e.g. walnuts, pecans and almonds)
seeds (e.g. pumpkin (pepitas), sunflower)

CONVENTIONAL (5 MINUTES)

1 COMBINE all ingredients together on a large platter.

Serve with unbuttered slices of some of the specialty breads, such as olive bread, fig and anise bread, apple and walnut bread, from your local bakery.

Melon Mates

For a minimum of work and a maximum of taste try wedges of unpeeled melon, such as pawpaw or watermelon, with a squeeze of lime or lemon to finish a meal.

Peeled and seeded melon halves make great containers for berries, drizzled with a little port.

Alternatively, serve cantaloupe halves with a dash of port as an appetizer.

Chilled Lychees and Honeydew Melon 'Bytes'

Canned fruit is useful to have on hand, as it mixes well with fresh fruit.

Try adding peeled and chopped honeydew melon to a can of lychees, with a sliver of ginger, and chilling for a colourful and cooling finish to the end of a spicy meal.

Seasonal Fruit 'n' Nut Platter

Summer suggestions

Serves 2

melon wedges, grapes, figs, strawberries,
walnuts, almonds, pecans, unsalted peanuts

Winter suggestions

apples, easy-peeling tangelos, bananas, pears,
chestnuts

CONVENTIONAL (5 MINUTES)

1 ARRANGE all the ingredients together on a platter.

Serve.

knife
plate
nutcrackers

HANDY MAN HINT *Do not drink anything you can eat whole — avoid fruit juices, eat whole fruit instead. The fruit has fewer kilojoules, more fibre and is more filling.*

FIT TIP *Grapes may be frozen successfully before serving.*

Dating Game

SERVES 2

2 large oranges, chilled
½ cup chopped dates
1 teasp cinnamon powder
½ cup flaked almonds
1 cup orange juice, chilled

CONVENTIONAL (5 MINUTES)

chopping board
knife
teaspoon
cup measure
2 serving bowls

1 PEEL the oranges, removing all the pith, and cut into 5 mm slices.
2 PLACE a layer or oranges in each bowl, sprinkle with the dates, cinnamon and flaked almonds. Repeat the layers with the balance of the ingredients.
3 POUR the orange juice over, and serve with yoghurt.

HANDY MAN HINT *Allow the dessert to marinate for 2–3 hours for a better flavour.*

VARIATION *Add 2 tablespoons liqueur (such as Grand Marnier or Cointreau) before serving.*

Dried Fruit and Nut Platter

SERVES 2

2 small pkts dried fruits (e.g. raisins or sultanas)
250 g nuts (e.g. unsalted peanuts or pecans, walnuts or almonds)

CONVENTIONAL (5 MINUTES)

plate
spoon

1 COMBINE all the ingredients on a large plate or platter, and serve.

HANDY MAN HINT

Add specialty fruit bread (without butter) to your fruit platter for extra carbohydrates.

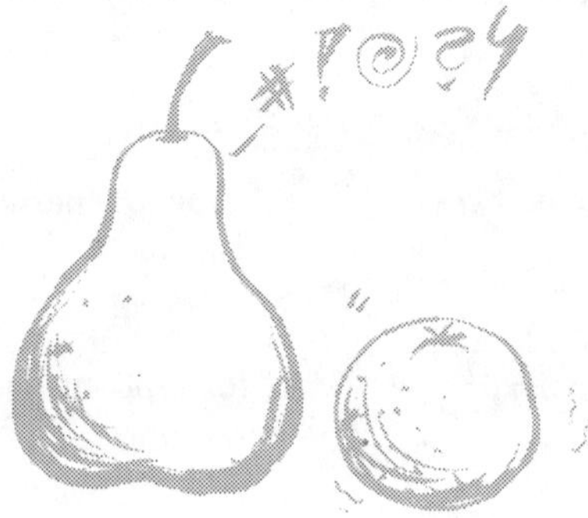

Goldfingers — Mood Food

SERVES 2

2 ripe goldfinger bananas, cut into 2 cm segments
1 orange, juiced
2 tablespoons honey
400 g low-fat banana yoghurt

CONVENTIONAL (5 MINUTES)

1 PLACE half the chopped bananas in each bowl.
2 DRIZZLE with orange juice and honey.
Serve with the yoghurt.

chopping board
knife
lemon juicer
tablespoon
2 bowls

HANDY MAN HINT *Goldfinger bananas stay gold even when cut, unlike other banana varieties.*

FIT TIP *Bananas are one of athletes' favourite foods — they are rich in potassium, fibre and carbohydrate, and are easily digested.*

VARIATIONS *Serve Goldfinger bananas sliced in a green salad, or on your favourite cereal.*

Pleasures of the Flesh — An Exotic Fruit Selection

Carambola: Green/yellow in colour with a clean waxy skin. Eat when green or yellow, on its own or sliced as a garnish for seafood or cheesecake. Good source of vitamin C.

Jackfruit: Light green in colour; it is ripe when the colour changes to light yellow, when it has a strong, pungent odour. Eat it raw or cooked, or in icecream. Excellent source of vitamin A and potassium.

Kiwifruit: Use when slightly soft to decorate cakes or cheesecake, or over icecream, or cut in half and eat with a spoon. Excellent source of vitamin C.

Nashi pears: Green/yellow or golden russet (brown speckled) in colour. Eat fresh as a dessert, or as part of a fruit and cheese platter. Excellent source of vitamin C and dietary fibre.

Purple and golden passionfruit: Choose smooth, dark-coloured fruit (avoid those that are excessively wrinkled). Delicious straight from the shell, or use in drinks or as a topping for cheesecake or icecream. Good source of group B vitamins and vitamin C.

Grown in Queensland, exotic fruits have a year-round availability, while being diverse in taste. This selection of fruit will cleanse your palate after eating Asian foods — without generating extra work!

INDEX